# GETTING IT RIGHT:

MILADY'S
SURVIVAL GUIDE
FOR COSMETOLOGY
STUDENTS

# GETTING IT RIGHT:

## MILADY'S SURVIVAL GUIDE FOR COSMETOLOGY STUDENTS

*by Alan Gelb and Karen Levine*

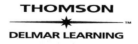

**THOMSON**

**DELMAR LEARNING**

Australia  Canada  Mexico  Singapore  Spain  United Kingdom  United States

## THOMSON

### DELMAR LEARNING

**Getting It Right: Milady's Survival Guide for Cosmetology Students**
by Alan Gelb and Karen Levine

**President, Milady:**
Dawn Gerrain

**Director of Editorial:**
Sherry Gomoll

**Developmental Editor:**
Judy Aubrey Roberts

**Editorial Assistant:**
Courtney VanAuskas

**Director of Production:**
Wendy A. Troeger

**Production Coordinator:**
Nina Tucciarelli

**Director of Marketing:**
Donna J. Lewis

**Channel Manager:**
Stephen Smith

**Composition:**
Type Shoppe II Productions, Ltd.

For permission to use material from this text or product, contact us by
Tel        (800) 730-2214
Fax       (800) 730-2215
www.thomsonrights.com

**Library of Congress
Cataloging-in-Publication Data**
ISBN: 1401817327

# Contents

# A LETTER TO THE STUDENTS

Welcome to *Getting It Right: Milady's Survival Guide for Cosmetology Students*. This book is a fun-to-read collection of practical, proven tips and hints to make the life of a cosmetology student easier and more productive. Hundreds of short tips are organized by category, making the information easy to find and fun to look through. Compiled from real-life experiences of students, teachers, and professionals throughout the United States, the tips are easy to digest and remember. They offer many not-so-obvious ways to make cosmetology school more manageable and preparing for licensure less threatening.

Congratulations on embarking on the exciting career of cosmetology!

—The Publisher

# ACKNOWLEDGMENTS

The authors and the publisher wish to express their gratitude to Dottie Soressi, the staff, and students of New York International Beauty School for their many helpful suggestions.

# Chapter 1

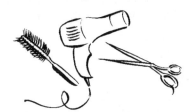

## GETTING STARTED

**H**ow are you feeling these days? A little overwhelmed maybe?

Well, that makes sense. After all, you've got a lot on your plate. You're enrolled in cosmetology school, you've got tuition to pay and a lot to learn, and there may be other commitments in your life that threaten to distract you from your goals. Do you have family to attend to? A boyfriend or girlfriend who wants more of your time? Are you juggling school and a job?

Whoever said life was easy? But the good news is that your life, right now as a cosmetology student, certainly isn't boring, is it?

Here you are, on the brink of this new chapter in your life, and you're excited, nervous, and hopeful all at once. Cosmetology may be a career you've come to only after a long period of confusion, insecurity, sacrifice, and who knows what else, but life is like that: hard times followed by good times, followed by hard times, followed by good times. Begin by taking a deep breath and telling yourself that these days in school are going to be the good times, full of promise and achievement.

Whenever you're feeling overwhelmed, tell yourself that others, not much different from you, have done it, so why not you? Better yet, read this book. It's filled with thoughts, feelings, and advice from cosmetology students just like yourself. We have gathered this information from all over the country and have organized it in a way to be most useful to you. Think of it as a resource to turn to when you're looking for ideas about how to make the most of your school experience.

## Going After the Dream

Before we get into anything else, let's start by having a look at the routes that some of your fellow cosmetology students have taken to get to the same place you're in right now.

**I tried different fields**—accounting, child care—but I decided that cosmetology is the easiest way to make money. As a customer, I've seen how much the stylists I go to make, just from me alone. I want to be getting that kind of money.

☙ **I'm having a change of career.** I've been a bartender and a waitress, but I wanted something with more freedom, more creativity. I want to do color. I'm really good at that.

☙ **I've been doing hair** since I was ten. First it was on dolls, then my mother bought me a head and I started practicing on that. I'd do my mother, my sisters, even my father. It was just a gift. I knew I was good at it. Now, I want to get my license and start my own salon, and maybe even start a school one day.

☙ **I've always loved to do hair.** I was always saying to my friends, "Look at your hair! Let me fix it!" They didn't mind. And I'm very social. I've worked in law firms and stuff, but one thing I've learned about myself is that I need to be able to talk to people during the day, have fun, and help people feel good.

☙ **I'm an artist** and I was supporting myself by working full-time as a salesman. My sister had a job at a salon, and some part-time work came up for an assistant on the weekends. She said to me, "Why don't you try it?" I figured, "Why not? It'll be a good way to meet girls." So I took the job and I really liked it. It was an outlet for my creativity and I was good at it. Now I want to get my license so I can have my own salon. I want to get heavy into editorial and have Ralph Lauren call me up and say, "Do my show."

☙ **I'm the youngest of three girls.** In first grade, I was already doing my sisters' hair and their friends' hair. I wanted to do a million different things—I worked in the hotel business, in the restaurant business—but I came back to hair because it's really my first love. But being in school has taken a lot of getting used to. I like hanging out with my friends and I don't have any time for that now. That first month, it was like, "What have I done to my life?"

☾ **I'm a barber by profession.** I've been barbering for 13 years and I own my own shop. But I want to get my license so I can open up a full-service salon. Plus, I've got two daughters and I'd like to be able to do their hair for their proms.

☾ **I've always loved doing hair** and I've been doing it all my life, but it's more than just about love. The thing I feel about cosmetology is that people are always going to need to have their hair done. There's always going to be work.

☾ **It's a family thing.** My mother and my sister both do hair. Mostly, I enjoy taking care of skin. I'm going to get my certificate in dermatology next.

☾ **I've got three little kids,** and as a working mother, I can't think of a better job. I make my own hours, work in my house, and am home after school. It's perfect.

☾ **I worked 23 years** as a manager for a cellular phone company. Then I got laid off. I always had an interest in doing hair, so I figured I'd try something nontraditional for a change instead of just looking for another job in the corporate world. I want to specialize in healthy hair. Healthy hair for African-American women. That's my dream.

## The Reality and The Dream

Dreams are wonderful things, but they have to coexist with reality. In the world of cosmetology, there are wonderful dreams to be pursued and wonderful realities to be discovered, but, as with every field, there are problems and pitfalls of which to be aware. Having a sense of these issues is very useful.

ↄ **I'm really excited** about the creative aspect of the work. I think that the idea of working in a career where I get to create beauty on a daily basis is the best!

ↄ **I like the idea** that I can be an entrepreneur in this business. I can rent a booth somewhere, for not a lot of money, and I can work for myself and build up a clientele. That, to me, is what's exciting.

ↄ **For me, the best part of this business** is that I can take my skills anywhere. I'm planning to live in London, Paris, Tokyo, and Sydney. I want to take my scissors and my blow-dryer and see the world.

ↄ **What races my motor** is making other people look good. Sometimes, I'll be sitting on a bus and I'll see somebody across the aisle, and I'll say to myself,

"I could make you look so much better, honey." It's a kind of power that I can't wait to let loose on the world.

﹏ **I'm feeling pretty up on the business**, but I have friends out there who tell me that I'll have to scale back some of my dreams now and then. I may find myself in a not very creative shop, doing the same old thing for the same old people, and that can be frustrating. But I'll cross that bridge when I come to it.

﹏ **I like people all right,** but I know that there are lots of not so great people I'm going to have to deal with. Clients, staff, my boss: I'm a little nervous about that.

﹏**I've heard that burnout is a big problem** in this field, particularly if I'm working for myself. I'm liable to find that I am unwilling to take a vacation, for instance, because that means lost income. Soon I'd be a workaholic, and how good is that?

﹏ **My aunt's a cosmetologist.** She says it's a great field, but it can be hard on your body. You've got to learn the basics of good posture and positioning and stuff like that.

The best way to make sure you strike a healthy balance between your dreams and the reality of life is by educating yourself. That's exactly what you're doing now since you entered this program. But to make the most of your education, you have to make sure that you're in the best shape—physically, emotionally, and psychologically—to *receive* the education. That's what this book is all about: helpful tips to get you into shape to *receive* your education. So let's get started with the business at hand.

## Self-image, Self-esteem, and Self-validation

We thought a good place to begin our discussion would be with the issue of image. Image is obviously a very important issue in the beauty field. People will be coming to you to improve or change their image. For the moment, however, let's look at *your* image. When you glance into the mirror, do you like what you see? Do you see an attractive, confident, connected person who stands a good chance of achieving success? Or do you see an unattractive, lazy, not-so-bright, not-so-special person who shouldn't even bother to try? Your self-image will have a lot to do with determining whether you make the most of this school experience or not.

Self-validation is an important issue as well. What does it mean to "validate" something? Well, think about it. You go to the mall and you have your parking ticket "validated" at one of the stores. That validation is a way to prove that you were there, being a good shopper, and your reward is free parking.

When we use the term "validation" with regard to personal growth, we're referring to something similar to the validation of the parking ticket. We're talking about "proof" that you exist as a significant person in the world. Too many of us look to other people for that validation. This need to have others validate us can cause us to become needy individuals, always looking on the outside for something that we would be better off finding within. Let's hear what your fellow students have to say on the issue.

ॐ **Let's face it.** We all start out looking for validation from our parents. They're the authorities that have been there and done that. But in my case, I had parents who were very withholding of their approval. They thought they could control me by withholding it, and so I got into this trap of always seeking that approval but never getting it.

ॐ **In our house**, dad was the big boss and ma was this submissive little mouse. Even though I love my mother and think she's a much stronger and braver person than she thinks she is, she frankly wasn't the world's greatest role model. I didn't learn until I was well into my teenage years that women could hold the power and that the only validation that really matters, in the long run, is the validation they bestow on themselves.

ॐ **I was married for 10 years** to a man who saw validation as something one got only by acquiring *things*. He was very successful financially and boy, did we have things in our lives: designer clothing, gold watches, fast cars, and so on. But something was missing. Even though I had fun with all the baubles and bangles, it ultimately felt empty and I realized I had to move on.

꒰ **I grew up in a family** where there was enormous emphasis on appearance. My mother had been a runway model, my sister is a model, and I was a teen model for a while, too. But as I grew older, I realized that the thing that gave me the most satisfaction in life was my relationships with other people. That's why I decided to go into cosmetology, because I felt I could get the kind of validation I was looking for by making *other* people look good.

# Searching for Success

Too many of us allow others to define success for us. Maybe your father thinks that the definition of a successful person is someone who makes $50,000 a year. Maybe your mother believes that a successful person is one who marries well. Do you have friends who tell you that the only way you can really achieve success as a cosmetologist is by owning your own business? All of these folks are entitled to their own opinions, but that's precisely the point: these are *their* opinions. You need to develop your own opinions about what success is and what you are willing to do to achieve it.

⌡ **The important lesson I'm learning** as I get older is that life is a matter of trade-offs. Maybe it doesn't always look that way, like when you see someone who appears to have it all: a career, family, friends. But for most of us, life is a matter of picking and choosing, one from Column A and two from Column B. Want a family? A couple of kids? Want to be involved with them and to be there when they need you? Then you may have to scale back on your career goals. You want absolute security and to know that when you're 60 you can retire and never have to think about money again? Well, if that's your goal then you may not want to go into your own business where there are so many highs and lows. You have to figure out what you want and then make choices to go with your decision.

⌡ **To be successful**, you have to first have a working definition of success. I've based my definition of success on my grandmother. She raised me, my brother, and our two cousins. She never made a fortune, but there was always food on the table and a roof over our heads. She was always kind to us and other people, and when she was needed, she was there. I think she was an incredibly successful human being.

⌡ **Who's to say what's success and what isn't?** Somebody might think that people who make a zillion dollars a year are successful. I think the postman who delivers my mail is a very successful guy. He likes everyone and everyone likes him. He'll retire with a government pension and he's in great shape from walking around the neighborhood in rain, snow, sleet, or hail. Now that's success!

🌀 **Your ultimate success and your values** are all tied up together. If you value nothing more than money, then you won't feel like a successful person until you've got a big fat bank account. For some of us, though, the thing we value most is the love of work. I've chosen to work in a salon where I might not get paid as much as I would in another salon, but I have more freedom to do what I do well. That counts for a lot, and if it means I have to make a little less to be able to enjoy that, so be it.

## Positive Thinking

Success, validation, and a good self-image all go hand-in-hand with a positive outlook on life. People who have a more negative orientation can achieve success too, but they have to work harder. Positive thinking is like rich soil; you can grow almost anything in it.

🌀 **I have a twin sister,** and it's funny, but the two of us are completely different. She sees a glass half empty while I see a glass half full. I remember once when the two of us pulled into a motel one summer weekend. We didn't have a reservation and we were lucky to find anything. So what did I see? A swimming pool (okay, so it was a little small, but it was wet), a room clean and air-conditioned, and a walk out to the beach. All Donna saw was a nicer motel across the street. That's just the way she is. Everything is seen through a negative lens.

꙳ **People who live in the land of negative thinking** sometimes slide right into an even more negative form of thought, which is the self-fulfilling prophecy. That means if you say to yourself, "I'm not good at memorizing things," you can actually convince yourself that you *can't* memorize things, and then your negative thought has become a negative reality. An alternative to that kind of thinking is telling yourself something like, "You're not world-class when it comes to memorizing things, but you can get better at it. There are mind tricks that you can learn. Anyone can develop a better memory if they set their minds to it."

꙳ **I learned the secret of positive self-thinking** from my father. He drummed it into me and my brothers and sisters right from the get-go. If we were having trouble with something, like learning to ride a bike or learning Spanish or whatever, he'd say, "You can do it. I know you can do it. So do it!" I carry those words around with me always: it's a voice in my head. In school, when we have exams coming up on something I don't feel confident about, I'll tell myself, "You can do it. I know you can do it. So do it!" It always works.

꙳ **Another kind of positive thinking** that I learned when I played basketball in high school is visualization. You *see* yourself doing something—like making a foul shot—and that seeing becomes doing. I've tried it when I've had to do some tough stuff in school and it helps me a lot. It got me through pin curls!

꩜ **I make it a point** to surround myself with positive people because I'm a positive person myself, and I don't want to be brought down by someone else's negativity. If I find myself around someone who is always griping and finding fault and making gloomy predictions about the future, I move on until I find someone else who is supportive and encouraging. The more positive thought I can bring to my world, the better.

꩜ **I combat negative thinking** with positive self-talk. This is something one has to learn. My minister taught me, but it's not a religious thing. It's simply a way of giving myself a pep talk. When I'm feeling down, I use it to boost myself up. I say kind, helpful things to myself, like "I'm a good person. I can do it. I can get beyond this." At first, I might feel a little self-conscious doing it, but soon enough, it gets to feel natural and then it gets to feel good.

꩜ **It's hard to think of a good reason** *not* to use positive self-talk. Lord knows, there are enough people out there in the world who are more than ready to provide you with negative input about yourself. You might as well be your own best friend.

꩜ **One thing I've learned to do** when I'm in a down mood is to head off really negative feelings at

the pass. If I start obsessing about my debts, for instance, I'll just say to myself, Stop Thought. It's like a
red flag that I hold up in my head. Sure, it's artificial,
but so what? It does the trick. It takes the wind out of
the sails of the negative thought, and, once I've done
that, I can clear the way for some positive thinking.

## Good Advice

Always be on the outlook for good advice. It can be
the key to helping you succeed. This advice can come
from anywhere—your parents, other family members,
friends, teachers, or other students or people in your
life like physicians or clergymen—but once you've
heard something that you think might be useful, try
not to lose it. You might want to pick up one of those
little memo pads to carry around with you so that
you can easily write down good advice whenever you
hear it. Here are some "life tips" from your fellow students that we thought deserved your attention.

〰 **I had a history teacher** in high school I really
liked. He always told us to have fun with whatever
we did. "Work is the highest form of play," he used to
tell us. Frankly, I was never 100 percent sure what he
meant by that until recently, when I got into cosmetology. I love what I'm doing. I feel the same way
putting my hands into a head of hair as I did when I
was four years old and I had my hands in clay. I look
forward to getting to school every day, which is not

to say that I'm not often tired or hassled or frustrated or whatever. But I love the essence of what I do, and that feeling gets me beyond the fatigue and whatever else threatens to drag me down.

☙ **A big part of growing up** is assuming responsibility, and I'm not just talking about becoming a parent or making a living or whatever. I'm talking about assuming responsibility for actions. If something goes wrong, don't try to blame someone else; accept the reality of what's happened and try to build on it.

☙ **I try my best** to eliminate the word 'failure' from my vocabulary. Instead, I approach every situation as a learning opportunity. If I 'fail' a test, that just gives me the chance to go back and relearn what escaped me in the first place. Failure is really just a state of mind . . . and not a state I choose to live in.

☙ **Look at the big picture.** Don't get bogged down in small things. My wife taught me this. When we first got married, I lost a camera. I was absolutely beside myself. I come from a family where if you lose an umbrella or a pair of gloves, you hear about it 10 years later. In her family, if you lose something, it's not the end of the world. "So you lost a camera," she said. "It cost $300. What's that going to mean over the course of your lifetime?" To me, that was an amazing concept.

☙ **Never underestimate the importance of other people.** For too long in my life, I was a loner. Loners have a mysterious air about them that some people find intriguing, but, in reality, it's hard to be a loner. Most things happen in this world because people realize that if they help each other, the road through life becomes much easier. That's why networking is so important and should be something you make time for all through your career.

↻ **My father always taught us** never to do half a job. No matter what it was—delivering newspapers or shoveling the path or washing the car—we had to put our all into it. Total commitment: that was the rule. And you know what? It was a good rule!

↻ **Look for the gift in whatever you do.** Let's say you go for a job and don't get it. Is it a disaster or an opportunity of some sort? Will it lead you, in fact, to a better job just a few weeks down the road? When you learn to think this way—that there's a gift to be found in every situation—it creates a feeling of hope that is very strong.

# The Seven Guiding Principles

Throughout this book, you will be reading tips about everything from test-taking to anger management to résumé writing. But the nitty-gritty advice that fills this book needs to be placed in the context of broader, more sweeping principles. We have developed these principles during the course of writing "Survival Guides" for professionals in a number of different fields. These Seven Principles are designed to help you determine what you value most in your life and how you can make room for these things you value.

Once you've read through these principles, it is important to do what you can to keep them in mind. You can put them on an index card that you carry in your wallet or your bag. If you want, turn them into a rhyme or a song, and chant them at quiet times or once a day in the morning or before you go to sleep. The goal is to develop a healthy perspective that will sustain you over the long run, that will help you have fun and enjoy life, and that will make you remember, at the end of a long day, what you truly value.

## Principle #1:   Become an Active Listener

Having decided to go into the cosmetology field, the likelihood is that you are a "people person" and that you've always been a good listener. If this is not the case, then you had better brush up on your people skills because as a cosmetologist, you will need them. In any event, when it comes to listening, in Chapter 7, you will find specific tips on techniques such as reflective listening, in which you reinforce what a person says by returning their words to them. As a guiding principle, however, we stress the importance of taking the time in a busy day to listen to others and to really hear what they have to say. Many of us are so overwhelmed by the demands and stresses at school, work, and in our personal lives, that we look for relief by drowning out our surrounding environment. That might mean walking around with headphones on, or, even more destructively, tuning out others by ignoring them. In fact, such actions intensify stress. You can get more stress relief by keeping open the lines of communication and enjoying your contact with other people.


## Principle #2:  Thinking Outside the Box

Life will be a lot more satisfying if you avoid the trap of conventional, unimaginative, stereotyped thinking. One of the challenges you may face as a cosmetologist might have to do with being asked to style hair in a way that does not appeal to your own sense of style. If such is the case, you will need to find ways to keep your creativity alive and fresh outside of your job and outside of the box. You may want to spend one or two evenings a week styling the hair of friends whose taste is as interesting as your own. Thinking outside the box will also help you avoid stereotypical thinking that has to do with body image. This kind of thinking is not only wrong and can get you into a lot of trouble, but also deprives you of really meaningful opportunities that you could be enjoying with others. Having a long-range view of things is another way of thinking outside the box. If you feel stuck in a rut, you need to keep your dreams alive by telling yourself that life is always filled with surprises that can take you to places you never even imagined.

## Principle #3:  Take Time to Figure Out What You Find Most Satisfying

Well-organized systems and routines can help ensure smooth sailing, but routines can also be overdone. When this is the case, you may begin to feel like a robot, moving through your day without really thinking about what you're doing.

Mihaly Cziksentmihalyi, Ph.D., Professor of Psychology at the Drucker School of Management at Clermont Graduate University, wrote an important book called *Flow: The Psychology of Optimal Experience* (Harper Collins, 1991), in which he presented an interesting study he ran with a group of adolescents. He gave them beepers that went off eight times a day over the course of one week each year. Every time the beeper signaled, they'd report in to him about what they were doing and how they were feeling about it. Among other things, he found that when these subjects were involved in an activity they enjoyed, they developed a sense of *flow*, a great feeling of energy that made them want to continue doing what they were doing and return to it whenever possible.

In Chapter 2, we will offer a tool and a technique to help you figure out just which activities give you a sense of flow. We will help you assess how you spend your time and how you feel about what you're doing. We will take you through your day—before, after, and during school—and we'll analyze where you feel most and least satisfied. This kind of honest assessment is a critical step you need to take before moving on to Principle #4.

## Principle #4: Create Time for the Things You Care About

The idea of shifting your time and energies to make room for the things you most enjoy may seem like common sense, but you would be surprised how few people actually live by this principle. Too many of us carry around a "can't do" attitude when it comes to changing our patterns. The good news is that most of us "can do," as long as we try.

Suppose you discover that you feel most ready to meet the day after you've had 30 minutes of quiet time to sit, read the paper, and sip your coffee. Or perhaps you can achieve a better mood for the day if you've been able to take a walk before going to school. You may learn that by shifting morning chores with your roommate or spouse, you can free up the time you need. Or you might decide to set your alarm a half-hour earlier every day.

With regard to school, you may discover that the best way to stay on top of your work is to deal with it as soon as it's assigned. Or maybe you do better when you let things sit a while and have deadlines breathing down on you. Whatever works. The key is to begin thinking about how you can best meet your needs because when your needs are met, you will be better equipped to meet the needs of others.

## Principle #5: Learn to Enjoy What's in Front of You

There is a Buddhist practice called "mindfulness" that teaches the value of focusing on what is beautiful in the here and now. Mindfulness urges us to live in the moment. Learning to develop this kind of vision is a huge help in clearing away the clutter of our lives.

How often have you found yourself thinking about everything other than what you are doing? You may be sitting in class and your mind is wandering to your bills, the bad wheezy sound coming out of your car, or a million other things. Think about what it would be like to really focus in on the moment and to be getting the most out of that class. Your teacher and your fellow students have a lot of worthwhile things to say. *You* have a lot of worthwhile things to say, too, and your active participation will go a long way toward making that class a better experience for everyone.

This practice of mindfulness can and should be used outside of school, too. When you're driving home, for instance, instead of thinking about your bills or the weird sound in your car or a school project coming due, think instead about how beautiful the light in the sky looks at that very moment or how peaceful the sound of the rain on your rooftop is.

## Principle #6: Learn to be Flexible

There is no such thing as a day that goes exactly according to plan. You have to learn to roll with the punches and the bumps and the trap doors that are always opening up all over the place. Cosmetology is a field particularly filled with the unexpected. Clients can either call at the last minute (or don't call at all!) to cancel appointments, or they may have "emergencies" when they simply have to see you. As part of a team, you may also be called on to fill in for someone else at the last minute. Even as a student, it's never too early to start thinking about how you're going to handle such situations.

Some people take change hard and think that they can get around it by setting down ironclad "rules" that others must follow. Such people are often seen as difficult, temperamental, in-flexible sorts who do not inspire affection or loyalty.

If you think of yourself as a kind of machine that is out there every day getting the job done (but, of course, you are much more than that!), then flexibility is the lubricant that will keep your gears in working order. Stress falls away in the face of flexibility and flexibility also softens the hard edges that can often be present in one's interactions with others. Flexibility will keep you from turning into a tight rubber band, ready to snap. Flexibility is like the elastic that allows you to retain your shape.

## Principle #7:   Prioritize

Once you know what you have to do, and what you *love* to do, it's time to prioritize and get rid of all the unnecessary, energy-sapping tasks that you dread. You'll be shocked by just how much choice you have when it comes to investing your time and energy. Remember to keep track of what you actually do with your time. Ask yourself:

✂ What do I need to do to take care of myself that absolutely no one else can do? For example, do I need to meditate at the end of a long day after having dealt with all the other things I've had to do? Or should I get together with some fellow students to tackle that subject matter that seems so hard?

✂ Which of my responsibilities can I put off for the moment, to be dealt with later with no harm done? What can I delay and what absolutely has to be done immediately?

✂ What am I doing that someone else could be doing for me? Could I ask my mother or my sister or my friend to take in my dog to the vet for her rabies shot?

✂ Is there something I can do in a different way to make my life easier? For instance, can I order my husband's birthday present over the Internet instead of going to get it in person?

Embodying these Seven Guiding Principles and letting them show you the way is not something that happens overnight. Some people take months, even years, before they can internalize them, and, even then, most of us have to be careful not to let old habits creep back into place. But we are not putting these principles forth as a way to create even more pressure for you. As time goes on, these principles will come to feel like second nature, and when you fully understand them and learn to live by them, you will appreciate and enjoy a quality of life you might never have experienced otherwise.

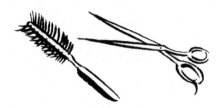

# Chapter 2

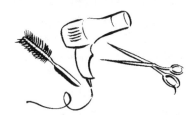

## STAYING ON TRACK

Generally, when people ask, "How are you doing?" most of us answer, "Just fine, thank you." We assume that there is little real interest in what was good or bad about our day. Such exchanges are just a way of being polite. But as the day goes on and we have that same exchange over and over again—"How are you doing?" "Fine, thank you"—the details of our lives often get blurred or even lost along the way. By the end of the day, we may not even be all that sure that things were fine, thank you.

In this chapter, we urge you to give some serious thought to how you actually spend your day. The best way to begin doing this is by keeping a record of how you use your time. Most of us spend 16 out of every 24 hours a day awake and active. (That's on a good day. Unfortunately, for some of us, the waking day may stretch out to 18 or 19 hours.) In those waking hours, some of what we do might make us feel great. We might be lucky enough to have been kept busy with activities that leave us feeling energized and happy, with that sense of "flow" that we cited in the first chapter. But, unfortunately, most people in the world have to spend some of their time, or even a lot of their time, doing things that they would rather not be doing, things that are boring or unpleasant or simply routine.

The truth is that most of us don't have all that much choice when it comes to doing what we have to do. With rare exceptions, we need to attend to the humdrum duties of life, whether it be paying bills, doing the laundry, going grocery shopping, cleaning up after the kids, or more of the same. But it is our belief that most of us can actually exert more control over our lives than we think we can. The key is to make a study of how we actually use our time and to keep track of how we *feel* about the ways in which we use our time. Once we've observed our patterns, we can begin to think about making some changes.

Think about how you're spending your time. As a cosmetology student, you're in a big crunch, aren't you? So many of you are doing double-duty, going to school while you hold down one or even two jobs. Some of you have a spouse and children to factor into the mix. This book is very focused on helping you make the most of your time so that you don't get strung out, burned out, or used up by all the demands being made on you. It's very important to step back and examine your life, because if you don't, these demands can get the best of you. Let's hear what some of your fellow students have to say about these demands and how they're coping.

❧ **There have been a lot of times** when I've just felt overwhelmed by school. Frankly, I've never been the world's greatest student. My sister, who's a year older than me, was always Wonder Woman when it came to school. She'd sail through every class and even if she didn't study for something, she'd still wind up getting an A. Me, I'm not like that. I have to work twice as hard as the next person just to keep my head above water. And when I'm working twice as hard as the next person, that doesn't leave a whole lot of time for anything else.

❧ **School doesn't go great with me** and my boyfriend. He resents every minute I'm not paying attention to him. He's such a baby . . . but a cute baby. He just doesn't understand that I've got so much at stake here. I mean, I've gone down two other career paths before this one. I don't feel like being a keypunch operator my whole life. Sometimes, I feel like I'm going to have to cut myself right down the middle to make this work.

❧ **I'm fine when things are going smoothly,** but half the time things don't go smoothly. The kids get sick or the dog gets sick or the car gets sick or there's a snow day or my mom needs me for something or who knows what? Then I start going crazy trying to live up to my responsibilities, and usually, I'll wind up having a fight with my husband and . . . well, you get the picture.

↩ **I'm the kind of person** who always takes on too much. I have a terrible time just saying no. I'll get a call from some P.T.A. mother who says, "We need someone to set up for the Halloween Party" and who do you think will always say, "Sure. Glad you called. Any old time." Even when I have huge school pressure bearing down on me. It's a sickness!

↩ **Sometimes I get so overloaded with work** and pressure and deadlines that I just go into a total turn-off mode. I can't look at a book or think about writing a paper or do anything more than just lie in bed and watch TV. Then I feel worse, incredibly guilty, I eat a lot of chocolate ice cream, and I hate myself.

↩ **I spend too much of every day worrying.** Instead of focusing in on what I have to do, I *worry* about what I have to do and whether I'm good enough to do it. I swear, I do such a number on myself sometimes.

↩ **I manage to get everything done** that has to get done, but I've always got this feeling nagging at me that there's got to be an easier way. Am I as organized as I should be? As motivated? Should I really have to be working this hard or am I just doing things the hard way?

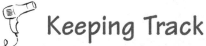

# Keeping Track

Now it's time for you to be the scientist and the specimen all at once. The idea is for you to develop a real awareness as to how you spend your time so that you can make sure you're working up to your potential, and that you're getting some pleasure and satisfaction in the bargain. The way to develop this awareness is by closely examining your day. Where do you go? What do you do? How do you feel when you do what you do? The pages that follow in this chapter make up a workbook of sorts. They will show you how to create a chart by which you can keep track of your day. The parts of the chart are as follows:

✂ Start/Stop/Total

✂ Activity

✂ Feelings

✂ Efficiency

✂ What's My Role?

You can easily create this chart in a notebook that you can carry around with you throughout the day. A small, spiral-bound pad will fit into almost any coat or jacket pocket for easy access.

Ideally, you will be creating a journal or log that reflects exactly what you do with your time in the course of any given day. This technique works especially well if you stay at it for a full week. Keeping track of your weekend activities and the feelings they bring out in you can provide an interesting contrast to your study of your workweek habits and feelings.

In your jam-packed days, it may be difficult for you to find the few minutes necessary to log your activities. When you've got classes to attend and projects to complete, and all the other demands that fill the rest of your life, it may not be easy to find the time to make notes about your feelings. The idea of this exercise is to make your life easier, not harder, so just do what you can to jot down your notes while the experience is still fresh. If you can, glance at your watch and make a mental note of the time you begin and end an activity; you can always jot it down later.

Some people find it easier to make notes on a small tape recorder or dictation machine, the kind busy executives use to keep track of their thoughts. Do whatever works for you, and do it as well as you can. Again, the idea is not to create another burden in your life, but to help you develop a powerful awareness about the way you spend your time.

## Start/Stop/Total

When taking stock of your day, you will need to be conscious of the clock, right from the moment your alarm goes off in the morning until you close your eyes at night. Think about the distinct areas into which your activities fall: classroom time, practice, studying, textbook time, and then the many non-school activities you spend time on like grooming, cooking, cleaning, shopping, and so on. Check the clock when you begin a new activity and jot down the time. Do the same when you finish that activity and before you move on to the next one. Don't neglect to factor in downtime like "hanging with friends" and the like. Whatever you do, don't worry about the "total time spent" until later. You don't need to burden yourself with adding, subtracting, and justifying yourself in the middle of a busy day. This is just straight numbers: five minutes making your kid's lunch, 10 minutes walking the dog, 25 minutes on the commute to school, and so forth.

↻ **It was really kind of fascinating** to do this Start/Stop/Total exercise. I could look at my whole day at the end, and when I was feeling overwhelmed, I could see how much I had actually gotten done.

↻ **As soon as I completed a week's worth** of Start/Stop/Total record-keeping, I realized how much time I was talking on the telephone. I just couldn't afford the time or the money, so it popped out for me as a place to make some changes.

## Activity

Once you start filling in your Activity chart, you'll be amazed at how many different hats you wear in a single day. You'll see yourself as a mother or father (took kids to dentist), as someone's spouse or partner perhaps (dinner at Julio's), as someone's child (took mom to the airport), as a friend (Sandy's birthday party), as an employee at your job, and, of course, as a student.

Keeping an Activity chart will also prove to you what a dizzying array of material you are studying as a student of cosmetology. You're learning everything from the structure of hair to the psychology of color. You're finding out all about client consultations, retailing, wigs and extensions, disorders of the scalp, hair relaxing, hair removal, and so on. A lot to learn. Your Activity entries will help you focus in on exactly what you're learning and the hands-on practice in which you are engaged. This will keep you from feeling that you are being bombarded by a huge mass of material.

Everything that is part of your day should find its way into your log. And remember, this is not something you're being graded on. This is for your eyes and your eyes only. You are the sole contributor and the only one who will be reading this. The goal is to learn about yourself, how you spend your time, and how you feel during the course of the day.

᷍ **When I started in school,** they give me this enormous textbook and I thought I was going to faint. Suddenly, I had to start reading stuff about electricity! But keeping tabs on my activities worked well for me. It showed me how much I was learning and I really liked that.

᷍ **The thing I really came to appreciate** when I started keeping track of my activities was how much I managed to get done. At the end of the day, I looked back on all that I had accomplished and I said, "Hey, girl. You take on a lot and you get a lot done. Husband, kids, job, school . . . good for you!"

## Feelings

Try to jot down your feelings soon after you have finished an activity. The closer you are to the feelings, the less inclined you will be to edit them, either consciously or unconsciously. Keep in mind that you do not need to write long, detailed notes here. A few words, if well chosen, will do fine. Begin by thinking in terms of "feeling" words: happy, sad, angry, bored, worried. Next, try thinking in terms of opposites—happy/sad, relaxed/tense, worried/optimistic, loving/angry, gentle/tough, energetic/tired, interested/bored—and judging to which of the two poles in each instance you feel closer.

It is also important in this section to gauge how much satisfaction you are getting out of your activities. Most of us have to do things that are not necessarily fun, but aspects of these activities can still bring us satisfaction. If, for instance, you are a very *tactile* person—one who likes using your hands, which you probably are given the fact that you have chosen cosmetology as your profession—then you probably get a certain sense of satisfaction from spreading a fragrant, luxurious emollient on a thick head of hair. If you are a people person—and again, it is most likely that you are if you have chosen to work in a people profession like cosmetology—then the time you spend studying up on client consultations may be the high point of your day. If you're not yet really sure what you like about this field, keeping this record of your feelings will help you identify the things that give you pleasure and may point you in the direction of more in-depth training in a certain area that interests you.

Remember not to think too hard and too long when you write down your reactions. Your gut response is probably the most reliable. Again, keep in mind that this log is for your eyes only, so don't worry about what others will think when you put down your honest reactions.

ᔐ **I enjoyed this part.** It reminded me of when I was a kid and I'd keep a diary and write my feelings down. When I'm running around a lot, just trying to get things done and to stay on top of it all, my feelings sometimes have to take a back seat. Doing this part of the log puts my feelings in the front seat, which is where they really belong.

## Efficiency

Did you ever go to someone who was great at cutting your hair but who couldn't get through the job without forgetting where he put some important tool or material? We figured you did. But you didn't hold that inefficiency against the person because he had talent, right?

Efficiency is *not* the most important thing in the world. We have all known people who are incredibly efficient and who bore us to tears. But it does count for something, particularly so in the life of a student. You don't need to be told that you've got a lot to keep on top of. Your coursework alone requires a lot of careful use of your time if you want to do your best. When you get out into the world, if you want to be a genius hairstylist who doesn't have to worry where you keep your tools because one of your many assistants can always supply you with what you need, that's fine. But for now, give yourself a break and organize your time and your activities as effectively and efficiently as you can. You'll save yourself a great deal of wear and tear if you do.

The point of the log is to look at the matter of efficiency—how best to use your time—and to see how you can bring it more fully into your life. Keep in mind that there may be instances in the log where efficiency does not really matter so much. For example, if you are looking at the time of day when you cook dinner, you may find that you don't necessarily choose to be as efficient as possible right then and there. While you might have a food processor that can do the job of chopping vegetables much faster than you, perhaps on that particular evening you are drawing a certain comfort from doing the task by hand, enjoying the feel of the vegetables and the steady slice of the knife. Maybe that is just the medicine you need to bring you down from a stressful day. So if efficiency does not apply to a given task, simply write N/A (not applicable) in your log. Otherwise, make an effort to rate your efficiency in any given activity on a scale of 1 to 5.

꩜ **This was a real eye-opener.** I saw myself doing things like making two trips to pick up stuff when I could have gotten it all done in one. Very interesting.

## What's My Role?

As we've suggested, over the course of 24 hours, you, like most other people in the world, play a variety of roles. You may be parent, child, spouse, partner, manager, mentor, or social worker. You name it. It is useful to think about which roles you most enjoy and which suit you best. For instance, even though you're a student, maybe you enact the role of a teacher now and then when you help a classmate understand something that you've been able to nail down. At another point of the day, maybe you're acting the role of an advocate or an activist, going to your school administrators on behalf of yourself and other students to register some dissatisfaction with something about your school. Maybe, for instance, there aren't enough lights in the parking lot and some of you feel nervous when you leave at night. Think about the roles you play and over the course of a given week, compile a list of them somewhere in the back of your notebook or pad. As you fill in your log, figure out the roles that you have been playing for each activity, but you don't necessarily have to write these down so close to the time of the activity. This category and the next—End-of-Day Analysis—can be filled in at the end of the day when you find some quiet time for reflection.

## End-of-Day Analysis

Now for the fun! The very last thing you do each day, just before you turn out the lights, is to analyze your log. This is your opportunity to learn something

|  | Activity #1 | Activity #2 | Activity #3 |
|---|---|---|---|
| Start | | | |
| Stop | | | |
| Total | | | |
| Feelings | | | |
| Efficiency | | | |
| What's My Role? | | | |

about yourself, and believe it or not, for many people, the results are genuinely surprising. Follow the steps below.

1. Begin by totaling the first column, Start/Stop/Total. Add up the total for each activity and note it.

2. Review what you've written in the Activity column and read across the row to What's My Role? Think about what your role has been in each activity and note it in the appropriate place.

3. When you've filled in the entire What's My Role? column, check back to the Feelings column and think about which roles you found most pleasurable or satisfying. Note as well those activities that you found least pleasurable or satisfying. Give yourself time to think about how you might rearrange your life to maximize your time spent in the pleasurable roles and minimize the time spent in those roles you do not enjoy.

4. Look back at your Start/Stop/Total column and match it up against the Feelings column. How much time did you spend doing things that offered you very little satisfaction? How much time did you get to spend doing the things you most love to do?

5. Think about what was most surprising in your log and make a note of it. Perhaps it was how much time you spent doing things that you genuinely do not enjoy. Or maybe—hopefully—it was the other way around. Maybe you're surprised by how much pleasure you took in learning some of the more scientific aspects of your coursework. Maybe you were surprised by how interested you were in a subject like nails or extensions.

6. Repeat this process every day for a week, each day with a new log. At the end of the week, go over all your notes, paying special attention to the End-of-the-Day Analysis. Give yourself ample time to think about what you are reading.

Again, the goal here is to reflect. Ultimately, you will want to find enough time in your life to do more of what you love to do and less of what you don't like to do. In order to achieve that goal, you will need to keep track of the Seven Guiding Principles:

1. Become an active listener

2. Think outside of the box

3. Take time to figure out what you find most satisfying

4. Create time for the things you care about

5. Learn to enjoy what is in front of you

6. Learn to be flexible

7. Prioritize

Keeping a log and being mindful of the Seven Guiding Principles is only one step toward making the most of your life as a cosmetology student. The next chapter will introduce you to the very important work of setting and achieving goals.

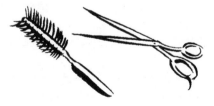

# Chapter 3

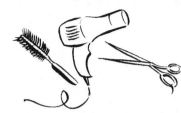

## THE GOAL ZONE

**Y**ou may already sense that cosmetology is a demanding profession. It isn't enough to be hard-working, talented, organized, ambitious, or any of the above. All of these elements are important, but no single one will ensure a successful career as a cosmetologist. The key to success in this field is to become a multidimensional person.

Now maybe that sounds a little scary. How do you know you'll be any good at being multidimensional? To this, we say, *stop worrying*. Worrying is one of those activities that will get you nowhere fast. The good news is that the qualities that will help you attain success as a cosmetologist are qualities that can be learned, and this book is one of the tools that will help you learn them.

In the course of this book, we present a lot of useful information on how to develop people skills. In any service profession, you will be dealing with a wide range of personalities. You may encounter individuals who are insensitive to your feelings or needs, and you will have to learn how to control your anger and frustration with clients, fellow workers, and management. Even if you own your own business one day, you will still need real people skills so that you can manage and motivate others, which can be even harder than motivating yourself and managing your own time.

As a cosmetologist, you will also need significant organizational skills to know how to plan your day, your week, your month, and your year. You will need to find ways to make room in your life for continuing education. The technological developments in the beauty industry are ongoing and the learning curve never straightens out.

As a professional in this field, you will need energy, stamina, and grit to help you carry your workload and to keep you fresh and active. You will also want to develop sufficient resources to keep from burning out on stress and overload. We will be offering good advice on how to protect your resources, and we will also be looking at ways to improve your learning skills so that you can digest and master all the material you need to know. Right now, however, we want to focus in on the very important skill of *goal-setting*.

The fact that you're sitting here right now reading these words means that you know something about goal-setting, even if you're not entirely aware of it. Still, you can't argue with the fact that you set a goal for yourself—to enroll in cosmetology school—and here you are, reading these words. That puts you leagues ahead of those individuals who haven't got a clue about their future and are waiting for inspiration to strike. Does that sound at all familiar to you? Did you spend time, before you got here, in that place? Congratulations, then, on meeting the goal you set for yourself, but there's something important that you should know about goals: they have a way of changing. That means that you have to continually examine the process of goal-setting to make sure that you are headed where you really want to go.

For most people, goals are closely connected to a concept of success. We touched on the issue of success in the first chapter, but we'd like to briefly revisit it here.

## The Fundamentals of Success

Success does not mean the same thing to all people. There isn't one way to be successful. Let's hear what your fellow cosmetology students have to say on this subject.

☾ **Some people will tell you that success** is making money, end of story. I don't agree. To me, it's a lot more than that. Am I a good human being? Do I do a good job? Do I work hard? Do people trust me and do I trust people? Money is nice, but you know what they say: it's only money.

↻ **Some people just hang in there** for years, and if they work hard enough and are patient enough, they'll achieve success. A lot of success is just about hanging in.

↻ **People say success** is all about who you know. Maybe that's part of it—I mean, connections don't hurt—but knowing people is also about being open to other people. If you're not open and you're not out there meeting people and networking and stuff, it's hard to be successful, particularly in this business where a lot of your clients come through contacts and word of mouth.

↻ **When I think of success,** I think of what's involved in surviving the tough times. Anybody can be a winner when things are going well. That's no challenge. It's when you're in a bad place—a crummy shop let's say, where people treat you badly—that your real stuff has to come out. What's that expression? When the going gets tough, the tough get going?

↻ **My dad** always likes to say that if you want to get by in life and make a success of yourself, you need a sense of humor. Don't let others drag you down. It's okay to laugh at yourself when things get crazy.

꿈 **I once had a teacher** who told us that the thing about successful people is that they see the big picture. They don't let details hang them up. They identify what they want and they go after it.

꿈 **My older brother** more or less raised us and he could be some pain in the neck. He was always yelling at us that we didn't work hard enough. We were lazy, he'd say, and we wouldn't get ahead in this world unless we were willing to put in the hours. Well, you know what? I think I've come to agree with him. There really are no free rides, and a lot of success has to do with just learning and practicing and working at getting good at something. For the most part, it's not about magic.

꿈 **I like to think** that almost everybody can be successful if they can figure out what their gift is. I think we're all born with some kind of gift, some special thing that maybe we haven't even discovered yet. Maybe we're musical or fast or strong or incredibly kind and patient or funny or beautiful or incredibly dependable. I don't know. All I know is that when one thinks of himself as being "ordinary," it hurts his chances for success.

꿈 **I don't know anyone** who doesn't want to be successful. Success is to life what sugar is to coffee. But the fact is that we don't all get to experience success, and even those of us who do sometimes have to wait a really long time before it comes. I've been an athlete all my life and so I was still really young when

I had to figure some of this out. When I lost a game, I had to learn not to beat up on myself. I really didn't help my chances of success by wearing myself out with self-criticism. My advice is, just tell yourself that everyone makes mistakes. Everyone goes through periods where they're not lucky and nothing's happening for them. Keep your good feelings about yourself alive by being good to yourself, and you'll survive until success is ready to visit you.

⌇ **My sister** is an accountant and she's pretty successful, but she's like a total workaholic. I worry about her because she doesn't even take time out to exercise or spend time with friends or whatever. I think that even if you become successful, you're not going to stay that way unless you make a point of taking care of yourself. You've got to take time out to enjoy life or otherwise you run the risk of becoming a burned out, one-shot wonder.

⌇ **To me,** success is something you can get good at, just like anything else. When you practice successful habits like good posture, good hygiene, dressing nicely, speaking so people can understand you, and stuff like that, it all works toward a positive self-image that creates a climate for success.

## Success Do's and Don'ts

You all know the expression, "Shooting yourself in the foot," don't you? It means finding ways to undermine your success. Why do people do this? They may have some very conflicted feelings about success. For example, in certain cultures, parents hope that their children will surpass them in terms of material success, while in other cultures, this would be frowned on. If you come from such a culture, you might be avoiding success for this reason. Or you might have fears of success because, deep down, you feel a certain sense of inadequacy that you've never dealt with and you're afraid that if you seem to be successful, you might somehow be "exposed." It is helpful to have some sense of the ways that we can encourage success in ourselves and the ways that so many of us discourage ourselves.

☾ **I've never been a great student** and I'm the first to admit it. It's just not where my head goes naturally. All through high school, the operative word with me was "procrastination." If I could put something off until the next day, that's what I'd do. Better yet, the next week. Better still, forever. It's a hard habit to break.

☾ **I've always identified with** Scarlett O'Hara in *Gone With the Wind*: "I'll think of it tomorrow, at Tara." Me, if I can think of something tomorrow, that's what I'll do. It drives my parents crazy. In fact, I've always been such a procrastinator that I actually had to get some counseling to deal with it, and now I know some good techniques. "Procrastination-busters," my counselor calls them. For instance, if I'm dreading something, like studying for a huge exam let's say, I'll find some little bitty part of the job that I can start with. Maybe it's sharpening pencils. Maybe it's organizing file cards, whatever. I just don't allow myself to sit there and be paralyzed.

♋ **All my life,** my parents were on my back about how I was such a procrastinator, how they had to light a fire under me to get me to do any little thing, and all that. It was such a drag. But guess what? I got out into the world and I've discovered that everyone procrastinates! Okay, maybe everyone doesn't procrastinate as much as I do, but it's not such a terrible sin. It's just a human quality. If you recognize it and deal with it, and you don't have to tell yourself that you're the world's worst lowlife because you do it now and then, okay?

♋ **For me,** the biggest trap has been perfectionism. I grew up in a home where everything had to be perfect. Every drape had to go with every piece of upholstery and every shoe had to match every dress and if you had a tiny little spot on something you were wearing the sky was going to fall down. Now that I'm an adult, I know that perfectionism is completely counterproductive to success. Feeling like I can never achieve what I hope to achieve is the opposite of motivation, and motivation is what breeds success.

♋ **I took a course** in human behavior in high school and we learned all about motivation. There are two types: extrinsic and intrinsic. Extrinsic motivation is when you get it from the outside like when your father offers to buy you a car if you get all A's on your report card. Intrinsic motivation is when you get it from the inside. You get all A's on your report card because you know how good it feels to do the best you can. Intrinsic is usually more long-lasting and effective than extrinsic.

☾ **Perfectionism** is a way of punishing yourself. Why? Because none of us is perfect. You could be the world's best at something and still have a really bad day. When you come down to it, aiming for perfection is a truly bad idea and can only leave you with the bitter taste of disappointment. Who needs that?

☾ **One of the definite "do's"** is to have a game plan. The short version of it is that if you've got a goal, then you need a game plan to reach your goal. Not having a game plan is like taking a car trip without a road map.

☾ **My dad** owns a liquor store so he's always telling me his theories about business. He says that anyone who owns a business or wants to own a business needs a business plan. It's the blueprint that gets you from here to there. It tells you what you should expect to make and what you have to spend. If you don't have a business plan, no one's going to lend you a cent. My dad says I should think of *myself* as a business, but instead of making a business plan, I should make a game plan that will tell me where I can expect to be in a year, in two years, in five years, maybe even in ten years.

♋ **My understanding** of a game plan is that it tells you what kind of resources and training you'll need to take you where you want to go. For instance, as a student, you need a game plan to help you figure out where you're going to get your tuition money unless mommy and daddy are just handing it over. But money's not the whole story. Your game plan should also help you figure out where you're going to find a quiet place to study, how you can balance your life as a student with a job, and so on.

♋ **My mom** owns a salon together with my two aunts and they say it's really important to think about a mission statement. The mission statement puts down on paper who they are and what their long-term goals are. It can be really helpful to see life in black-and-white that way.

♋ **Here I am** in cosmetology school, and believe me, I'm no kid. It's taken me a while to get to this place. That's why I felt it was really important to make a mission statement for myself. I wrote it down on a 3 x 5 index card and I had it laminated, no kidding. Listen, I've got a lot of distractions in my life—two kids, an ex-husband who doesn't like to live up to his responsibilities, a mother with chronic health problems—so it's really easy for me to get waylaid from my goals. The mission statement keeps me on track.

## Goal-Setting

Okay, you've got a clear enough concept of success, or at least what success means to you. You understand that success can be undermined by certain negative habits and behaviors like procrastination and perfectionism. You also understand that success can be promoted by certain good habits and behaviors like creating a game plan or writing a mission statement for yourself. Now's the time to look at goal-setting, what it's all about and how best to go about it.

☺ **There are goals** and then there are goals. In other words, some of your goals are going to be short-term—you can achieve them tomorrow or next week or a couple of months down the road—and other goals are there for the future. Owning your own business, for instance, is a long-term goal for a lot of us in this field.

☺ **When I think of** long-term goals, they're not so much about *things* as they are about *feelings*. For instance, one of my long-term goals is to feel financially independent and secure. And I have a goal to be in a long-term relationship with someone I love and to have children. When I really think about what my goals are, one is them is definitely to feel really good about myself. Now some of these goals may take a very long time to achieve, even a lifetime, but hey, that's life.

☺ **Setting goals** is a great idea, but like most other things in life, there's a right way to go about it and a wrong way. The wrong way is to set goals for yourself where you're continually falling short of them. That's going to leave you feeling disappointed and even discouraged, which is counter to the whole idea of goal-setting. What I've learned to do is to break down my goals, even my short-term ones, into smaller "goal-units" that I feel confident I can accomplish. For instance, when I decided to enroll in cosmetology school, I was really worried in the beginning because I'd been out of school for quite a while and I was never such a great student to start with. But I decided to break the experience down into a bunch of short-term goals. So instead of focusing on the long-term goal of getting a degree or getting licensure, which frankly intimidated the heck out of me, I've focused on short-terms goals like getting a project done or passing an exam.

ॐ **Setting goals is fine,** but don't you think they have to be thought out? You don't just say, "I'm going to do so-and-so." You need to figure out exactly what you have to do in order to get so-and-so done. You've got to ask yourself questions like, "What skills do I need to reach my goal?" "Do I need to take more classes?" "Can I find a coach or a mentor to help me?"

ॐ **Goals and dreams** are two different things. I once had a dream to be a ballet dancer but I broke both my legs in an automobile accident. End of dream. Goals should be things that are possible for you to achieve. If you've got chronic back problems, for instance, you might not want to become a hair stylist who's on your feet all day. That's a no-brainer. If you find it painful to talk to strangers, you might not want to become a hair stylist whose job involves talking to strangers. That's also a no-brainer.

**Goal-setting never ends.** It's not as if you get to the top of the heap and then you're finished; no more goals. Just look at any amazingly successful person and you'll see that they're always raising the bar higher.

## Dealing with Disappointment

Goals are important, but just as important is the way you cope with not meeting your goals. Your capacity to deal with disappointment will prove key to how successful you are at getting through life.

**Life is full of landmines.** I remember one Christmas, I was working at this small ad agency in our town, doing mostly clerical type stuff, and I was let go. My employers felt really bad about it, but it couldn't be helped. They had to cut payroll. Well, I carried on like it was the end of the world. I mean, fired? At Christmas? What could be worse? Well, guess what? A couple of weeks later, my sister-in-law was in a terrible car accident and had to be in rehab for close to two months. That's worse. And that was my lesson: whatever happens to me, something worse is happening to someone else, and if I fall short of a goal I've set for myself, I just move on. That's life.

**Disappointments can lead you** down streets you wouldn't find yourself on otherwise. Take my cousin. She was working at a salon that went under. It was no surprise because it was not a well-run business. But she wasn't motivated to go out and find another job until this happened. It took her a little while but then she found this awesome job at this day spa that she's been at for the last six years. The bad news turned into good news.

☾ **My parents** always taught us that if we've been disappointed in something, it's important to look at the situation and to see what we did right and what we did wrong. Everything is a learning experience, they always told us. There's no such thing as failure. There's just good stuff and bad stuff, and we've got to learn from it all.

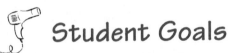 # Student Goals

We will be discussing your goals as a student in depth later in this book. But for now, it makes sense to give an overview of your goals as a student and how you can best work toward these goals. We polled your fellow students on the subject.

☾ **I want to be the best** I can be. This is *my* education. I'm paying for it with *my* money. I'm not doing this to make someone else happy. I'm doing this for me.

☾ **I never miss a class.** In high school, I don't want to tell you how much I cut. Not here. There's too much to learn, and if I don't learn it, I can't do it.

☾ **I don't want to sound** like Little Miss Perfect or anything, but I think one of the things to strive for as a student is to carry myself like a professional. I've already been out in the world—I worked in a child care center for a couple of years—and I'll be the first to admit that I had to learn a thing or two about professionalism. Now, I find myself looking at kids in my program who come in late two classes out of three or who gab with their pals instead of paying attention to the instructor, and I think to myself, "Okay. You've got a lot to learn, too."

☾ **One of my goals** as a student is to really get used to being a student and to realize that, to some degree or another, I'm going to be a student for the rest of my life. The cosmetology industry is always changing: new trends, new technology, new products. To stay on top of it all, I've got to read the industry magazines and books and go to trade shows and advanced classes. I can't just sit there, and I figure that while I'm still enrolled in school, I might as well get into the habit of doing more than less.

☾ **I've always been** kind of shy in the classroom, so one of my goals as a student is to speak up when I don't understand something. I ask a lot of questions but nobody seems to mind.

## Knowing What's Out There

As a student of cosmetology, it's great for you to have big goals. If you want to imagine yourself owning a salon or a day spa or half the world one day, go right ahead. But it's also very useful and interesting to know what other kinds of opportunities are out there in the field, and to keep these in mind when you're setting your goals.

↪ **What's really struck me** so far as I get to know this field is how many different ways I can use my knowledge. I mean, I went into school thinking I was going to be working behind the chair for the rest of my life, but it's totally not like that. I can go in a dozen different directions.

↪ **I like all the technical stuff**—the salon skills and all—but I think down the road, I'd be a really good manager, too. I'm bossy in a good way: at least that's what my brothers tell me. I seem to be able to get people to do what I want them to do without a lot of trouble.

↪ **I love everything about haircolor!** Coming into this field, I remembered that I was pretty good at art in high school. I never pursued it because my parents thought it wasn't a "real" career, so I went to a business school and got a job in a big corporation as an administrative assistant and hated it. Now that I'm in cosmetology school, I'm completely fascinated by everything having to do with mixing colors and formulas and all that. And I'm really good at it!

↪ **I'm thinking about** maybe specializing in texture services. The idea that I can take some chemicals and totally change the way a person looks is a lot of fun. And I hear it pays really well, too.

꩜ **You never know** what you're going to get into when you come into this field. My sister became a cosmetologist about five years ago, and she decided that she loved working with wigs. She's always been a great caretaker of people and she really was drawn to the work of helping cancer patients. She's set up her own little studio to specialize in this at a big salon and is doing really well.

꩜ **I'm going to have a hard time** deciding what to do because there's so much I like. I love skin care, for instance, and the idea of working in a day spa really appeals to me.

꩜ **I'm going to be frank:** I'm in this for the money. As much as I can get and as fast as I can get it while still staying legal. One of my teachers said he could tell I had a killer instinct when it came to sales. He said he bet I could sell ice cream to Eskimos or something corny like that. Anyway, he suggested that I keep the idea of retail in mind. Maybe I'd want to become a retail specialist. At first, I thought that was like a glorified sales clerk or something, but the more I hear about it, the more I think it's a good way to get what I'm looking for: a lot of money fast.

꩜ **I don't care** what I do: hair, nails, skin. All I know is that I want to work in a day spa. Why? Because I love the feeling of the environment and because I want to be able to get incredible discounts on all those services!

꩜ **I want to own a salon.** That's my dream. I'm willing to deal with bills, payroll, taxes, the whole enchilada. I just want to make it the best salon in the world.

☾ **I think it would be pretty cool** to be a product educator. I'd get to travel, always meet new people, and there's a lot of forward advancement. I'm a really good communicator, so I'm thinking seriously about it.

☾ **Nail art, baby!** That's for me. I love the idea of being able to go over the top creatively. I can't think of anything that's more fun and to be paid for it? Go on!

☾ **I was always really good** in science in school. In fact, I was thinking about becoming a medical technician at first. But since I've been in cosmetology school, I found out that there's this job called a cosmetic chemist. I would do experiments and research to create new products. I could work for a cosmetics company or as a consultant to a bunch of companies. Doesn't that sound like an awesome job?

☾ **I'm a stargazer.** Always was, always will be. If there's a star coming out of a stage door, I'm there, waiting for a glimpse. So I've got my heart set on doing something with my skills in show business: a makeup artist, a session stylist who works on photo shoots and stuff, maybe a job doing hair on a sitcom or a soap opera. Who knows?

☾ **One of the things** I think I'd have fun doing, in addition to a regular job in a salon or whatever, is being a platform artist. I'd like doing demos at trade shows. I think it would be really interesting.

✂ **I've always been a good writer.** Maybe I'll decide one day to be a writer in the industry. There's always a need for books, articles, videos, and stuff.

As you can see, there are many opportunities in the field of cosmetology. Identifying your interests and setting goals for yourself is the route to a satisfying and productive long-term career. For now, however, let's zero back in on the skills you'll need to succeed as a student.

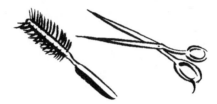

# Chapter 4

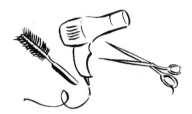

## BRAIN POWER

**W**ell, ladies and gentlemen, here we are, back in school again and. . . . Wait a minute. What if you never liked school to begin with? What if school always left you feeling intimidated, inadequate, and misunderstood? School was okay if you were one of the smart kids or if you were popular or athletic, but if your talents weren't exactly jumping up and down, then it could be a pretty painful place. And now that you're back, is it going to be any better this time?

Oh, yes, ladies and gentlemen; it's going to be much, much better. You can count on it.

Think back to the last chapter and what you read about goal-setting and motivation. The best kind of motivation was the *intrinsic* sort where the desire to achieve came from within you, not from what your mother or your father or your grandfather had to say. This time, because you've got that intrinsic motivation, you're ready to devote the energy, the hours, the money, and the passion to this pursuit. As you'll see, motivation is a force that can totally transform the school experience. Keep this formula in mind: School + Motivation = Achievement. There's nothing to stop you now.

But you still may be holding over feelings of inadequacy from your earlier school experiences and we don't want to see you sabotaging yourself in any way. We want you to be able to give yourself your very best shot this time, and to that end, we are going to focus in on ways that you can also learn to become a better learner. We all have reservoirs of brain power that we can tap into. That is not to say that we are all geniuses or that we're going to give the wealthiest or brightest person we know a run for his money, but, if we understand how our minds work, then we can make the most of those minds and do better than we've ever done before.

## The Big Brain

What weighs approximately three pounds and is made up of billions of cells so tiny that 30,000 of them would fit on the head of a pin? No, the answer is not some cute little extraterrestrial. The answer is the human brain, that amazing organ that acts as the conductor for everything that goes on in our bodies.

The brain tells our eyes, ears, nose, mouth, hands, and feet exactly what to do—laugh now! Cry! Blink! Snap your fingers! Wriggle your toes!—and it also regulates all of our basic life support systems like breathing, sleeping, feeling, and so on.

Those teeny-tiny cells we mentioned above are called neurons. Chemicals called neurotransmitters, which move from one neuron to the other and activate electrical impulses, stimulate the neurons. When you learn something—like how to give a basic shampoo, for instance—a particular group of neurons is activated and certain perceptions, memories, thoughts, and feelings are brought into play. So when you learn to adjust the temperature of the water spray when giving a shampoo, your neurons store away the information that any spray that is too hot or too cold is likely to disturb the client. Similarly, the neurons will store away the information that the smell of burning hair means trouble. Listen to those neurons, ladies and gentlemen; they're worth paying attention to!

As humans, our ability to store this kind of information is the key to our success as a species. We can't swim like sharks, jump like kangaroos, or fly like eagles, but we can learn much. Pianists can memorize entire concertos, athletes and dancers can remember extremely complicated physical routines, and cosmetologists can remember a staggering amount of information that has to do with the needs of their clients.

The human brain is a tough thing, encased in a hard protective shell called the skull, but it also needs to be taken care of. Substances like alcohol or narcotic drugs can dull or even destroy the brain. Certain psychological responses to stressful situations like anxiety or depression can also impact on brain function, causing forgetfulness or other impairments. As a cosmetologist, you will often be exposed to stress, whether it is in the form of long hours, demanding clients, environmentally unsound conditions, or demanding bosses, and you need to be sensitive to how that stress is impacting on your thought and reasoning processes.

## Intelligence

What can we say about intelligence? Some of us may have more of it than others and some of us may be able to access what we've got more readily than others. What's interesting, however, is that there is no one kind of intelligence. More and more, researchers are rejecting the idea of the I.Q., and are turning away from the standardized testing that suggests that all intelligence can be measured on a numerical scale. While it is true that certain kinds of intelligence can be assessed in this way, there are other forms of intelligence that do not lend themselves to such assessment but that are every bit as real and important.

It is very important for you, as a student, to understand that there are varied forms of intelligence because in your earlier days as a student, your areas of intelligence might have been discounted and your self-esteem might have been bruised.

In 1979, the world-famous educator, Harold Gardner, Ph.D. of Harvard University, presented his Theory of Multiple Intelligences. Gardner's theory stated that there are Seven Basic Intelligences, which can be present in an individual in various degrees of strength (*Celebrating Multiple Intelligences*, 1994 & Armstrong, 1994). These Seven Basic Intelligences are:

1. Word Smart (Linguistic Intelligence)   the capacity to use words effectively, whether oral or written.

2. Logic Smart (Logicomathematical Intelligence) the ability to use numbers effectively and to reason well.

3. Picture Smart (Spatial Intelligence)   the capacity to accurately see the visual-spatial world.

4. Body Smart (Bodily-Kinesthetic Intelligence) the ability to use the entire body as a means of expression, as well as to use the hands to make or alter things.

5. Music Smart (Musical Intelligence)   an aptitude for appreciating, creating, and/or expressing yourself through music.

6. People Smart (Interpersonal Intelligence)   the facility to know how to "read" other people and interact effectively with them.

7. Self-Smart (Intrapersonal Intelligence)   the capacity to see and know yourself well, and to reflect meaningfully on your experiences.

As we said, all of us have one or more of these kinds of intelligence, and each of these intelligences is just as important as the next one. Recognizing this information is vital to building up your all-important self-esteem.

↻ **All through school,** I always thought of myself as being the dumb one in the class. But I was—and am—a terrific dancer. I might have even been able to make a career of it if I hadn't damaged my tendons when I was a kid. Now I realize that, as a dancer, I had more than my share of bodily-kinesthetic intelligence. I wish I had known about this multiple intelligences theory earlier in my life so I could have felt good about myself. But now I can see, from the way I move around in class, and how good I am at holding tools and stuff, that my "gift" comes in very handy in this line of work.

↻ **Throughout my life,** I've had to deal with learning issues. I was a really late reader, math terrified me, and when it came to Spanish, it was unfathomable to me. I thought of myself as being pretty hopeless, and there was a long period where I just drifted. But then I started giving haircuts to my girlfriends and it felt really right. We would talk and laugh, and I would listen to them when they told me how they wanted to look and what kind of impression they were hoping to make, and I realized that I was really good at listening. In fact, I'm a great listener and I get along really well with people. I think that means that I'm high in social intelligence, and you know what? If

I had to pick one kind of intelligence to have, that would be it. I'd rather be good with people than with words or numbers any day!

☾ **Knowing about this theory** of multiple intelligences allows me to look at myself in new ways. I can see my strengths, and I have to say that I think I've finally chosen the right path for myself. I've got a lot of visual intelligence—I even thought about being a graphic artist when I was younger—and a good deal of body smarts and people smarts, and given the fact that I'm really good on the guitar, I've got musical intelligence as well. I'm not great at balancing my checkbook, but I figure if I make a lot of money one day as a stylist, I can hire somebody to do that.

# Remember This

One of the most important functions of the brain is to remember and retrieve the data it stores. Our brains reminds us to eat when we're hungry, to sleep when we're tired, to find our way home in our cars, to take our pills, to pick up our kids at the child care center. There are some things that our brain might be less on top of—Great-Aunt Minnie's birthday, for instance, or the mayonnaise that we were supposed to buy when we went to the supermarket—but we can live with such shortcomings. As cosmetologists, however, the memory lapses we suffer can cause embarrassment, anger, and even the loss of a client. If Mrs. Jones shows up and you have neglected to write down her appointment and are unavailable to her, she will probably be hopping mad and may never return to the salon. And if you do something like this more than once, word begins to spread that you're a bit of a flake. Talented, yes, but are you really worth the trouble?

Now, if you're one of those people who could never memorize the capitals of Idaho and Nevada, and can't remember if President Jefferson came before or after President Adams, then you may already be approaching the issue of memory with a sense of dread. Some part of you knows that you could forget to write down an appointment and you don't want to screw things up for yourself. But the good news is that there are ways to enhance your memory. Let's hear how some of your fellow students have gone about it.

✌ **I discovered an incredible way** to boost my memory: always keep a pencil or pen and paper handy. Seriously, I'm really into making lists. My memory was never so great to start with, and now, as a student, I have a whole lot of other things pulling at my concentration like having to make a living and dealing with my two kids. So I never go anywhere without my organizer and post-its for my dashboard.

✌ **I rely on all the usual things,** like to-do lists and calendars and stuff, but I've also discovered this other great trick. If I have something that I cannot, under any circumstances, forget—like calling my mother-in-law to wish her a happy birthday or sending in money for a class trip or something—I'll leave a message for myself on my own phone machine. It's pure genius!

🌙 **Whatever I have to remember** I say five or six times in a row. *Pick up Ned at the airport at 7. Pick up Ned at the airport at 7. Pick up Ned at the airport at 7. Pick up Ned at the airport at 7. Pick up Ned at the airport at 7.* Of course, if anyone heard me, they'd think I was a complete nut case, but the fact is, that's how I get something to stick in my mind.

🌙 **I make up songs** about stuff. For instance, one of the first things we had to learn in school were the bones of the face (two nasal, two lacrimal, two zygogmatic, two maxillae, one mandible). So I made up a song about them to the tune of the Beatles' "When I'm Sixty-Four." *Two nasal bones, two lacrimal, two zygomatic bones. Two maxillae and one mandible . . . these are all the bones of the face.* Is this going to win me a Grammy Award? I highly doubt it, but it got me to remember this stuff!

🌙 **There are things** called *mnemonics* and you've got to know how to use them. They're memory aids—a way to boost your brain—and you probably learned some of them when you were a kid. A famous one is HOMES, which is a way to memorize the five Great Lakes with each letter of HOMES standing for one of the lakes (Huron, Ontario, Michigan, Erie, and Superior). I make up mnemonics like that. For instance, if I need five things in the supermarket like bread, eggs, apples, milk, and salt, I'll make up the mnemonic BEAMS. I did something like that when we had to memorize the three phases of the growth cycle of hair. There's the anagen, or growth phase; the catagen, or transition phase; and the telogen, or resting phase. So naturally I took Catogen, Anagen, and Telogen and came up with CAT.

↻ **The older you get,** the more of a struggle it can be to remember stuff. For me, cosmetology is a second career—I worked in sales forever—and I have to work harder at memorizing things. So that's exactly what I do: I work harder. I give myself practice memory drills all the time, not just for my coursework but also to remember things like the names of other students in my school. I just want to keep stretching my memory to keep it limber. It's almost like doing calisthenics of the mind.

# The Care and Feeding of the Brain

Let's not forget that the brain is a part of our bodies and like the other parts of the body, it benefits from tender loving care. We rub oil into our skin, get a massage for our aching backs and necks, a manicure for our fingernails, and a pedicure for our toenails, but what exactly are we doing for our brains? Here are some tips from your fellow students about ways to coddle your gray matter.

☾ **Rest.** Rest, rest, and more rest. Sleep. Lots of sleep. Our brains take in so much on a daily basis, particularly in this high-tech world we live in where they are bombarded by images from all kinds of media—including the computer—that they absolutely hunger for some peace and quiet at the end of the day. So take a nap, do some meditation, listen to some calming music with headphones, put a cool compress over your eyes, and recharge.

☾ **I like to do crossword puzzles,** acrostics, and hand-held video games. These are all ways I have of keeping my mind limber. Other people might say I'm simply upping the ante on what my brain has to process, but to me, it feels more like an energizing thing, the way my body feels when I do ten laps in the pool.

☾ **Aerobic exercise** helps your brain work better, too. Jogging, swimming, biking, aerobic dancing, walking: they all improve oxygen flow to the brain and the brain is grateful for it.

☾ **I've read that** a balanced, low-fat diet is not only good for your heart, but helps with your brain function, too.

☾ **You've got to make sure** you're getting your proteins. Proteins are what the neurotransmitters use for building blocks, and the way to get these proteins is to make sure you've got enough chicken, fish, meat, beans, seeds, and nuts in your diet.

🌀 **My grandmother** used to serve a lot of fish all the time. I hated fish back then, but she always told us that fish was "brain food." We laughed at her—we were sure it was an old wives' tale, up there with wearing garlic on a braid around your neck or whatever—but guess what? Current research shows that fish really is a kind of brain food. Fish that is high in fats—like tuna, salmon, and sardines—apparently really does boost your brain power.

🌀 **Don't go loco** with the cocoa. Or the coffee or the tea or the colas or anything else that's high in caffeine. Caffeine may "perk" you up for a while, but the brain knows better, and when it catches on to what you're trying to pull, it'll crash.

🌀 **Stick a cucumber in vinegar** and you've got a pickle. Stick a brain in alcohol and you've got a pickle. No joke.

🌀 **We humans are born** with two eyes, two arms, two legs, two kidneys, two lungs. There's some insurance in having two of each of these. But we've only got one brain. So why would anyone go motor biking, skiing, bicycling, or in-line skating without a helmet? It's crazy.

## Think About It

Most of us are born with perfectly functional brains, thank goodness. It's how we use them that can be a problem. We have to learn how to think, and for some of us that process may not kick in so effectively until we are fully mature. The kinds of thought processes we're talking about involve logic, deductive and inductive reasoning, critical thinking, and creativity.

## Logic

Training your mind to have a certain standard of discipline can be a helpful way to face the world. Some people, of course, do just fine playing the role of the featherbrained gal or the silent hunk who don't think very much, but you might want to choose a sturdier role for yourself, like the person who comes up with solutions and solves problems. Problem-solvers are always going to be in demand in any field, any job, any time, any place.

What will distinguish you as a problem-solver is the degree of logic you bring to your thinking. Logic is a certain kind of ordered thought that is strong and that can support your actions. One type of logical thinking is called *deductive reasoning*. In deductive reasoning, the conclusion you come to is true because the underlying basis, also known as the *premise*, is also true. Consider this example:

Premise  Brushing machines, scrubs, and harsh mechanical peeling techniques can be injurious to skin with many visible capillaries.

Premise  Mrs. White has skin with many visible capillaries.

| Conclusion | Do not use brushing machines, scrubs, or harsh peeling techniques on Mrs. White. |
|---|---|

Another type of logical thinking is called *inductive reasoning*. Here, the conclusion may often be true but you have to check to make sure. Consider this example of inductive reasoning:

| Premise | Mrs. Jones' mother suffers from noticeably thinning hair. |
|---|---|

| Premise | Thinning hair is often hereditary. |
|---|---|

| Conclusion | Mrs. Jones will develop thinning hair. |
|---|---|

Now, there's a good likelihood that Mrs. Jones' hair will thin, but inductive reasoning prevents us from reaching such a conclusion, doesn't it? After all, there are exceptions to the rule of heredity and Mrs. Jones might be such an exception. For all you know, Mrs. Jones is not even her mother's biological child. The point is that you have to think. That's what the brain is there for.

Logical thinking also allows us to differentiate between fact and opinion. Claiming that olive oil works well as a hair treatment is, for instance, an opinion, and one that is shared by many people, if not whole cultures. But if you were to research this claim, you might not find any hard evidence or facts testifying to any proven merits of olive oil as a hair treatment. In an industry in which there is so much marketing and so much hype, your ability to distinguish fact from opinion will be important in helping you maintain your integrity as you market to your clients.

## Problem-Solving

There are two kinds of people in the world: those who think and those who depend on others to do their thinking for them. In our society, the vast majority of people fall into the second category. They are consumers of ideas, put to them by television, radio call-in shows, the Internet, and so forth. The rate at which this group is growing is alarming, particularly when you consider that many media outlets like newspapers, radio, and television stations, and magazines are all coming together under the umbrella of a small number of media conglomerates. The ability of a few to control the thinking of many thus becomes a real danger to democracy.

People who fall into the first category—those who actually, genuinely know how to think and who realize that most problems are open to examination and are subject to creative solutions—are always going to be in demand. They are problem-solvers who provide society with what it needs most: good ideas.

We spoke to students like yourself to see how they viewed the issue of problem-solving. Here is some of what they had to say.

✂ **People don't expect** cosmetologists to be problem-solvers. It's like, "Great minds do not go into cosmetology." But I think that's dead wrong. Some of the smartest people I know are in cosmetology. These are people who know how to run a business, who know how to get along with other people, and, for all of that, who know how to solve problems. Okay, maybe there are more pure geniuses in microbiology than in cosmetology, but wherever there are problems—and you're going to find out how many problems there are in this field—you need good minds to come up with solutions.

𝒞 **There are certain myths** about intelligence and what makes a good problem-solver. To me, Myth #1 is that if you've got a college degree, you're smarter than somebody who doesn't. That's so bogus. A piece of paper does not make you smarter than somebody else, and when you think of the way so many people go to college today, cutting classes and hitting beer parties instead of the books, the fact that they have a piece of paper that says they graduated from State U. means to me that they paid college tuition and not much else.

𝒞 **Sometimes, I've got to laugh** at how much we've become a society that runs after "experts." Your dog has an accident on the carpet and you're dragging her off to some expert on the mental health of poodles. I think we all need to become more of the experts ourselves. Since when did going to an expert to solve a problem become better than solving it yourself?

𝒞 **I'd say problem-solvin**g starts by identifying your goals and projecting ahead into the solution, even if it changes in the process. Ask yourself how you'll know when the problem is solved. What do you think the solution might look like? Be clear about your objectives. What are you trying to achieve? What are you trying to avoid? What do you want to get rid of and what do you want to hold onto?

↻ **You've got to be able to** define the problem. What is it? What are its main characteristics? Try to describe it, even writing down a paragraph on it if you can. Try to explain it.

↻ **Keep the blinders off.** Too many of us plow straight ahead in life without seeing as much as we could be seeing. Don't be so linear. Look around you, above you, below you. You never know where a good solution is going to come from.

↻ **I'm a big believer** in brainstorming. If I've got something that needs figuring out, I'll pick up a pizza and get some of my friends to come home with me. We'll sit around with the pizza and some wine, and if necessary, some brownies until we come up with some good ideas and possible solutions.

## Critical Thinking

Situations present themselves to all of us, and we have to be able to look at them critically and make wise decisions. For instance, if we go to a party with someone, and that person gets drunk and then offers us a ride home, we have to be able to look at that situation and judge it on its merits. Do we allow ourselves to be driven home by someone who gets behind the wheel after having had six shots of bourbon? Of course not. We call a cab. This ability to analyze a situation and take appropriate action is called *critical thinking* and it depends on logic, reasoning, and the ability to separate fact from opinion.

☾ **I'm always struck** by how little critical thinking most people bring to certain situations. For instance, we had a class the other day that involved a lot of chemicals and tools and what have you, and this one student brings in a pizza! Don't you think she would have had enough judgment to realize that pizza and perm solution don't go together?

## The Creativity Factor

Creativity is an important issue in the life of a cosmetologist. Generally, we can assume that you have not chosen this field so that you can do the same two or three hairstyles over and over again, day in and day out. One reason you probably chose this field was that you saw it as an outlet for the creativity that you feel has always been so much a part of you. However, one of the problems you may encounter in this field is that there are fewer opportunities for genuine creativity than you might have hoped for, and you are indeed doing the same styles day in and day out. In such situations, until you can find a different situation that better suits your need for a creative outlet, it is important for you to keep your creativity alive and well. Creativity, after all, is like health: you need to protect it, preserve it, and foster it. The more you use your creativity, the more it grows.

What exactly is creativity? Some people define it as the ability to take existing objects and to put them together in different ways so that they can serve a new purpose. Other people use a broader definition of creativity: the ability to generate new and useful ideas and solutions. Let's have a look at how your fellow students view the issue of creativity.

ᔕ **The best way I've found** to make creativity happen is through sharing ideas. I zero in on people who I think are truly creative and I recharge with them. We'll have coffee together or we might go to a museum or a movie or a concert, and we'll talk about what we've seen or heard. It gets the creative juices going.

ᔕ **One way I try** to keep my creativity alive is by having relationships with people outside the world of cosmetology. I have friends who are artists, writers, musicians, teachers, a biologist, and a close friend who's an attorney, and from each of them I get a different view of the world. I think it's very important to get away from the "world as cosmetology" view of things.

ᔕ **My older sister** is a photographer. She's really good and has had a bunch of one-woman shows. When I've asked her how she stays creative, she tells me that she's got to "surprise her mind." That might mean taking a different route to work some mornings, or eating dessert first or having breakfast for dinner. Pancakes in the evening will make the whole day feel different, and when the day feels different, it's easier for creativity to make an appearance.

☙ **I like to watch children.** The beauty of children is that they're not afraid to try things. They look at a problem and they're not worried that their solution is not going to work. They just go ahead and let it rip. Picasso said that every child is an artist, and I think he was right. The problem is how to remain an artist after you're all grown up.

☙ **Make time for creativity.** Sure, it takes more energy to be creative than not to be, but it's also more energizing. Sitting around watching TV is not going to energize you, you know that. But throwing a pot or knitting a sweater or having some fun with watercolors is going to energize you plenty.

☙ **I keep a journal.** It's where I focus my thoughts and jot down all kinds of ideas, crazy as they may be, without feeling the need to censor myself. I write in it every night before I go to bed, just for a few minutes. It's enough to stay in touch with that part of me that too easily can get lost in the shuffle of life.

☙ **A valuable lesson** I learned about creativity is that I shouldn't judge myself harshly. I took a drawing class because I wanted to be able to see people with new eyes. Our instructor, who was great, told us in the first class not to criticize ourselves. "That's just a way of censoring your creativity," he said.

☙ **For me, creativity is** very connected to the experience of the senses. Listening to music, looking at art, inhaling the scent of lilac, tasting a fresh fig: any of these can let loose a creative impulse in me.

💫 **Learn to recognize** your "creative time." We all walk around with a certain internal biological clock. Some of us are night people; some of us are morning people. If you're a morning person, don't sit down to write a song or a poem at midnight when you're ready to fall off your feet. Go with the flow of who you really are.

💫 **When you come down to it,** creativity and education go hand in hand. If you feel like you're getting stale and old hat, find a new way to do something. There's so much out there in terms of educational opportunities that there's no excuse not to do that.

💫 **Creativity is something** you can really work at, and to a certain extent, learn. At least you can learn ways to grow it. There are many good books on the market about creativity and many places where you can do workshops on the subject.

Now that we've looked at ways that the brain works, let's turn next to the issue of how we can develop good habits so that the work of the brain is made easier.

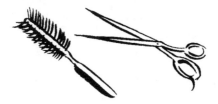

# Chapter 5

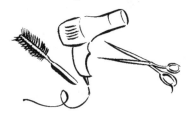

## STUDY SKILLS

**H**ave you ever heard your teacher say, "Let's recap?" He or she is referring to *recapitulation*, one of the most important steps in the learning process. To recapitulate means to summarize or review briefly. When we review material, we plant it more deeply in our brains. So let us take a moment to review, or recap, some of the more important concepts we've talked about so far in this book.

✄ *Self-validation and self-esteem.* These terms refer to a sense of feeling good about who you are, which, in turn, can lead to a better chance of realizing your goals.

✄ *Positive thinking.* A natural or learned way of reinforcing self-esteem.

✄ *Success.* A goal that is determined by personal values, societal values, or some balance of both.

✄ *Motivation.* The fuel that energizes you to achieve your goals and that inspires you to strive for success. Motivation can be extrinsic (external) or intrinsic (internal).

✄ *Procrastination and self-sabotage.* Destructive behaviors that detract from your chances of success.

✄ *Multiple intelligences.* Different but equally valid ways to think.

By recapping, we reinforce what we have learned and make it more solid. Now that we've recapped some of the highlights of what we've covered in this book up to now, we can move on to the topic at hand, which is how to develop powerful study skills.

Learning to be a good student is no different than learning to be a good driver or a good golfer or a good cook. You learn a set of good habits—don't tailgate, don't slice to the right, don't oversalt—and the more you learn and practice, the better you become. In this chapter, we will be looking at good study habits and hearing from your fellow cosmetology students about what works for them.

## A Quiet Place to Study?

People will tell you that if you want to succeed as a student, you have to carve out a quiet place for yourself where you won't be disturbed. A library is perfect, these people will assure you.

Don't believe a word they say.

Different people learn in different ways and these different ways are called learning styles. Your learning style will determine what kind of studying works best for you. There are three basic kinds of learners: *visual learners* who like to see what they have to learn; *auditory learners* who need to hear what they have to learn; and *tactile-kinesthetic learners* who choose to touch what they have to learn. Look at how some of your fellow students identify themselves.

## Visual Learners

**I'm a visual learner,** big-time. I've got to see what I learn. In other words, I never met a graph or diagram or chart or illustration I didn't like.

**As a visual learner,** my idea of horror is looking at 10 pages of text without any illustrations. Now maybe some people would say, "Oh, you're not too bright. You need to go back to the kiddie encyclopedia." To those people, I would say, "Oh, you're not too bright. Visual learners are just as smart as any other kind. We just learn differently."

**Being a visual learner,** I always take a seat in the front row. The only way the material can really be driven home for me is if I can see my teacher's face and body language.

☾ **Color** pushes my learning buttons. I have this whole system of using color markers to highlight my readings and notes and stuff. Pink means it's super-important material, yellow is very important, green is if I have time, and so on.

☾ **I am such a visual learner** that sometimes I'll even use this technique they use in ad agencies and on films and TV called storyboarding. It's basically telling a story in pictures. So if I have a demonstration I have to do in class, I'll draw myself going through the steps. It's a little weird maybe, but it helps me a lot.

☾ **Visual learners** generally have to study in quiet places. That's just the way we're made.

☾ **I always make flashcards** for myself. They worked for me when I was 10, and they work for me now when I'm 29.

## Auditory Learners

☾ **I learn by listening.** Being given a bunch of handouts doesn't do me a whole lot of good. I need to hear the words. Classroom discussion reinforces the learning for me.

☾ **One thing I've come to know** about myself is that it's easier for me to remember something if I can hear it. I'm the kind of person who can pick up Portuguese by listening to tapes in the car. So I decided to tape all my classroom stuff and that way, I can listen to it in the car to and from school or on my headphones if I'm jogging.

❦ **You know what helps** me a lot? Reading the textbook out loud. If I hear something, I can remember it better. So if you find yourself sitting next to me on a bus, you might catch me mumbling about microdermabrasion or alkanolamines or alopecia or what have you. It can get pretty funny.

❦ **I find that** if I can make up some kind of musical jingle to reinforce what I need to learn, it helps, like diseases of the scalp set to "Old McDonald Had a Farm." *Androgenic alopecia eei-eei-o.* Okay, so maybe it'll never make the countdown, but it works.

## Tactile-Kinesthetic Learners

❦ **We're the group** that learns by moving, doing, and touching. We go right to the "Touch-Me" part of the museum. Obviously, cosmetology is a very tactile field, so we're right at home here.

❦ **Lots of us** were labeled ADD—Attention Deficit Disorder—when we were younger. Now it's become clear how biased so many of those judgments were against people with our learning styles. We learn when we can move. If we can't move, it's hard for us to learn. There's nothing wrong with us.

❦ **I know this** about myself: as a tactile learner, I need to take a lot of breaks. I have to stand up and go to the refrigerator and the bathroom and stretch and throw a ball to the dog. That's the way I learn and the fact is that I actually learn fine. I'm a perfectly good tactile learner. End of story.

꩜ **Because I have to move** a lot, I do my reading on a treadmill. There's a little contraption that I bought where you can rig up a kind of shelf to attach to the treadmill to rest a book. It's a system that works fine for me.

꩜ **Any kind of movement** helps me when I'm studying, so one thing that I've learned to do is to hold something in my hand that I can move around and manipulate such as a piece of clay or a smooth rock. Just a little thing like that goes a long way. Even chewing gum helps.

꩜ **Sometimes, I'll go to a café** or a bookstore that has a café in it to do my studying because the feeling of movement around me is almost as good as moving around myself.

## Setting Up a Study Space

What you've just read indicates that the kind of learner you are will determine the kind of study space you're drawn to. Not too quiet for some people, not too loud for others. Whatever the volume turns out to be, there are sure to be other issues regarding your study space. Consider the following responses.

꩜ **I need a door.** I need to be able to close that door. Without a door, I feel naked and exposed and completely open to any kind of distraction. Now maybe that's my problem, but the fact is, it's *my* problem.

↪ **When I decided to go back to school,** I told myself that I could work just fine on the kitchen table, the way I used to when I was in fifth grade. But I'm not in fifth grade anymore—in fact, I have a kid in fifth grade—and I need my privacy. I need a place to keep my things and to know that little hands are not going to be messing up my papers. Is that so much to ask?

↪ **I made an office** for myself out of a closet— literally, a coat closet—right off the kitchen. I'm still in earshot so I can troubleshoot problems as they come up, but I'm just far enough away to have some feeling of distance, even if it's only an illusion of distance.

↪ **My dream office** has a big desk, a great chair, good light, a nice view, and a bed to flop down on. My real-life office, on the other hand, doesn't even have a window. The desk is a piece of junk, and there's no bed. But I do have the two most important things: the great chair and the good light.

↪ **Even though my office** is this tiny little ugly room down in the basement, I've managed to make it into a place that feels okay for me. I've put up a lot of photos of the kids and drawings they made for me and a snake plant (what else is going to grow in a basement?) and this little babbling desk fountain that my husband got me when I started school. I love that thing.

☾ **You've got to set up** your systems. Figure out what you're going to need and try to have it in place right at the beginning instead of having a crisis every time you realize you don't have something and you've got to run out to the store. You need calculators, pencils, pencil sharpeners, file folders, magazine files, a dictionary. All that stuff.

# Day or Night?

Once you have a good understanding of your particular learning style along with a good place to study, the next thing is to figure out the best time to get your work done. To determine this, it helps to have a sense of your *biological clock*. This clock is a small group of brain cells that send and receive signals to and from other parts of the brain and the glands. A person's biological clock is not present at birth; newborns have no sense of a daily rhythm. During the first year of life, however, the biological clock kicks in, and as the years go by, it becomes increasingly sensitive to certain factors, chief among them, daylight. Some people have biological clocks that are so sensitive to light that when the light is diminished, as in autumn and winter, they may become sleepy or depressed and may even need light therapy (see more about this in Chapter 8, Holistic Hints). Most people do not function as well at night as during the day, although a poll of adults questioned indicated that 10 percent to 15 percent of those asked classified themselves as early birds, 15 percent to 20 percent called themselves night owls, and the rest fell somewhere in between. Disturbed daily rhythms caused by poor sleep will upset a person's metabolism and appetite, and can lead to headaches, comfort eating, and excess weight. It is important, therefore, to understand your biological clock and to work with it.

↭ **I'm a night person.** If I try to get up early in the morning to get some work done, I'll spend half my time walking around like a zombie looking for the coffee filter. I'd always rather stay up late than get up early.

↭ **I always thought of myself** as a morning person until I had my kids. Now, even though I'm often exhausted at night, I'll make myself stay up late because I know that at night, after the kids have gone to sleep, that's the only time I can be sure I'm not going to be interrupted. I let my phone machine pick up any calls—people know not to call me after a certain hour anyway—and I just plug away until one or two in the morning.

↭ **I can block out** just about anything. In fact, my father says that I have raised blocking out things to an art form. I always carry my work with me wherever I go. If I go to the dentist or I'm sitting on a train or whatever, I'll use that time for studies. Let me tell you, it adds up!

↭ **More important** than the time of day you like to study—morning, noon, or night—is that you keep a consistent sort of schedule. If you study in the morning one day, the evening another day, an hour here, or four hours there, you don't really work up a routine, and routines help you get through something like studying.

☙ **If you're a slow starter,** you should know that about yourself. Factor in an extra half hour for warm-up time. Maybe you need coffee, a look at the paper, some yoga stretches: whatever gets you going. If you proceed at your own speed, your mind and body will be grateful.

☙ **My kids know** that they do their homework and mom does her homework at the same time every day: right after dinner. Then we usually get back together later in the evening for some cookies and milk and maybe play a couple of hands of cards or watch a little tube.

☙ **Naps are important.** They refuel you. A 10-minute nap, or even a five-minute one, can keep you going for hours. Try it.

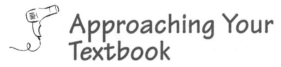 # Approaching Your Textbook

Your cosmetology textbook may look to you at first like a great big monster. It approaches 1,000 pages in length. Yikes! Maybe it scares you silly. But it doesn't have to. Do you remember when we talked about procrastination? We said that it was helpful to divide up big jobs into smaller units. The same approach makes great sense with your textbook. When you look at it for the first time, you might be thinking to yourself, "I have to know *that*?" Clearly, such a prospect can feel overwhelming. On the other hand, the idea of reading and digesting individual chapters is much less intimidating. And keep in mind that your textbook was designed to be a user-friendly object. You just have to know how to use it.

↻ **The first thing I do** when I start a chapter is to look at all the headings and other organizational clues. Just about everything you have to know that's important is signaled. It's either in bold type or italics, or there are bullets next to them (the little round black dots that are easy for your eye to pick out).

↻ **The thing I like about textbooks** today is that they take the visual learner into account. I can remember back in high school having these old textbooks with very little illustration. But our cosmetology textbook is filled with pictures, charts, tables, and so on.

↻ **I always go to the end** of the chapter first, to the review section, to get a good idea of what's really the most important stuff in the chapter. Then, when I've got that overview, I'll go back and start reading because the plan of the chapter is in my head.

↻ **Before I read one word** of a chapter in the textbook, I do a survey of the whole chapter. I look at all the titles and heading and pictures. I get a sense of what the architecture of the chapter is all about.

☙ **I had a teacher** in high school who told us that when we read something, we should always be asking questions as we go along. What's this all about? What is the author trying to say here? What's the main idea of this paragraph? What are the supporting examples?

☙ **I mark up my book** a lot when I read. I use highlighters and put stars next to important stuff. Let's just say I customize it.

☙ **There's a myth** that you've got to read every word of a textbook assignment. Not so. There are often little "extras"—sidebar columns, for instance— that have information that may be interesting but that isn't crucial. The main ideas make themselves known. They're usually right out there, in big bold letters, where they can't be missed.

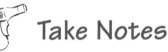 ## Take Notes

In the course of your time as a cosmetology student, you will need to take notes about what your instructor is saying. This may be a skill that you never mastered in your earlier school experiences. You may have sat through classes where other students were writing away and you may have wondered what the heck they were doing. But note-taking will prove to be a significant skill for you as a cosmetologist, both now and in the future, when you will be involved in continuing education, attending workshops and trade shows, and will want to take note of what presenters have to say. Let's hear what your fellow students have to say on the subject of note-taking.

☾ **If I know I'm going to be** in a lecture-type situation or somewhere where I'm going to have to take notes, I'll sit right up front. That way, all the distractions are literally behind me.

☾ **It's a job, taking notes,** and like any job, you need to have your tools ready. If you're cutting hair, you've got to have a comb and a scissors. If you're going to be taking notes, you need a pen and paper and some bottled water so you don't have to get up to get a drink if you're thirsty and stuff like that.

☾ **Usually, when someone's giving** a lecture or a talk or some kind of presentation, they'll structure it with a beginning, or introduction; a middle; and an end, or summary. The introduction and summary are really important. The introduction lets you know where you're going. It orients you for the whole thing, so you've got to pay careful attention to it. That's not the time to check your phone messages or ask your friend how his date was last night.

☾ **One thing that I had to learn** about note-taking was to make it short and sweet. At first, I'd try to get every word down. That's impossible. The idea is to put the instructor's words into your own words. You want to understand what she says, not duplicate what she says.

☙ **If the instructor is** any good at what he does, he's going to cue you as he goes along. He'll say things like, "First" or "Next" or "For example." You've got to learn to pick up on the cues. Some instructors will even cue you really heavily, saying things like, "This is important. You've got to know this" or even, "This is going to be on the test." I love instructors like that.

☙ **The summary's** going to put it all in a nutshell. Get it down because that's the stuff you really, really need to know.

☙ **I used to be** a doodler. No more. I know they say that some people concentrate better when they doodle, but I don't buy it. When you're paying total attention instead of doodling, you're getting a lot more out of what you're hearing.

☙ **Whatever the instructor emphasizes,** I'll emphasize in my notes by putting a big green star next to it with my highlighter. Or if she gives an example, I'll put a big X for eXample next to it.

☙ **I always try** to write as legibly as I can, which takes some effort for me. But if I don't, then I waste a lot of time on the other end trying to decode what I've written.

☙ **Somebody taught me** this trick of abbreviating. Like instead of writing "and," you can make a plus sign (+). Or, if it allows you to write faster, you can leave out letters of recognizable words like writing *csmotlgy*, for instance, instead of writing out *cosmetology*.

☾ **If you have any questions** at the end of the presentation, don't be shy to ask them. That's the time for it.

☾ **Sometimes, when the instructor is** summing up at the end, I'll look around and everyone is packing up and stuff. I want to say, "What's the rush? Don't you realize you're missing some of the most important stuff?"

☾ **I always try to go over my notes** right after the presentation to make sure that I got it all and that I can understand what I wrote down. It's good to do that while the material is still fresh in my mind.

☾ **A really good strategy** for note-taking is to use the two-column format. You make one column wide and one narrow. In the narrow one, you jot down the important thoughts you pick out as you review all the main ideas and important facts in the wide column. For instance, if your wide column is full of facts and information about pH, you might want to stick an important point like pH 7 NEUTRAL in the narrow column.

☾ **It's generally a good idea** to use an outline form when you take notes. You don't have to make it literally an outline with Roman numerals and A, B, and C and all that. But you should at least use indentations so that you can see, at a glance, the relationship of the main ideas to the supporting points.

# Testing, Testing . . . 1, 2, 3

Some people are afraid of spiders or cats or heights or flying. It may be difficult, but if you suffer from such fears, you can more or less arrange your life to avoid them. You can stay away from the woods where spiders lurk and you can take trains instead of planes and you can resolve never to go skydiving or hot air ballooning if heights are an issue. But one of the most common fears is also one of the most difficult to avoid. That's the fear of taking tests. It is so strong that it can make those who suffer from it physically ill, and it can undermine an otherwise rewarding school experience. For those who suffer from test anxiety, all the telltale signs are there: the sweaty palms, the clammy pallor, the butterflies in the tummy. Testing anxiety can wreck a school career, but the good news is that *it can be overcome*. A little behavior modification can deal decisively and constructively with most cases of test anxiety.

☾ **I've always hated tests.** Even my driving test was, like, torture. But, in recent years, I've figured out some things about test-taking that help. First of all, I tell myself, "It's only a test." Even if it's a huge test, a licensing exam, let's say, what's the worst that's going to happen if I fail it? I'll have to take it again. Big deal. You have to put a test into perspective. Even the big, big tests like the licensure examination are still just tests. If you fail, it doesn't mean you're a useless person. It just means you're human.

✆ **You have to get yourself** physically prepared to take a big test. That means, the night before and certainly in the morning, you don't want to drink a lot of coffee or cola or eat junk food. Instead, you want to calm yourself with some wholesome carbohydrates like brown rice or fruits and vegetables. Listen to some Mozart or Bach or some of that nice calming music with a Celtic feeling. And most of all, get a good night's sleep. I know that's easier to say than do, but it will really make a difference.

✆ **I think it's useful** to understand that test anxiety doesn't have to be eliminated entirely. That anxiety can help you get "up" for the event. You know how if you're about to go on a stage or out onto the playing field for a big game, you've got the adrenaline flowing and it boosts you up onto another level of focus? Well, test anxiety can be like that, too. It's up to you to judge when that anxiety becomes counterproductive.

✆ **Some of your anxiety** can be taken down a few notches if you know that you've prepared yourself well for the test. And I don't mean just studying. I mean going further back and seeing to it that you've been to all the classes, you've kept up with the work, and you didn't have to cram the night before. A lot of times, anxiety becomes overwhelming because it's fed by the guilt you feel from having procrastinated and not doing what you should have.

↺ **Lots of us** have formed groups for one thing or another in our lifetimes. Maybe we've been in support groups for some problem, like debt or overeating, or maybe we've been in something like a book group for fun. Don't forget that the good, supportive feeling we get out of a group can work for you in a study context, too. Try getting together with a couple of other students and form a study group that meets regularly, especially when an exam is coming up.

↺ **If ever there was a time** for positive self-talk, it's in the testing situation. That's when a lot of your negative internal voices come out, the ones that say things like, "I always screw up on tests" or "I'm the dumbest one in the room" or "If I mess up on this, it's over." Control those negative thoughts with the "*stop thought*" approach—when you feel them coming on, literally say to yourself, *stop thought*—and replace them with positive thoughts, like "You've really prepared yourself well for this and you should do fine" or "You did well on the last test, so you'll do okay on this one."

↺ **Don't look around** the room and compare yourself with others. Mind your own business. That way, you won't distract yourself.

↺ **Practicing relaxation** should be an ongoing activity. But it's one of those things that we all have to get good at. I use what they call guided imagery. I'll imagine myself in a place that I really love and that I find totally relaxing, like the front porch of a Victorian-style bed and breakfast on the beach at Martha's Vineyard. As I put myself there, I'll feel a lot of the tension ooze out of me. The other thing that's good to try is called progressive relaxation. Start at your toes and say, "Relax your toes." Work your way up your body, inch by inch, and say, "Relax your knees," "relax your belly," "relax your chest," and so on. The higher up you go, the better the relaxation payoff. But, again, it takes practice.

↶ **Always make sure** you give yourself plenty of time to get to your test. You don't want to come rushing in, out of breath, having stressed yourself out to the max looking for a parking space or whatever. Adding stress to stress is the last thing you need.

↶ **I'm a pretty social person,** but I always sit by myself when I'm about to take a test. I don't want any distractions and I certainly don't want to pick up on somebody else's anxiety. Anxiety is contagious!

↶ **If you've got an exam** scheduled, ask your instructor well in advance if you can take a practice exam. That's a great way to build up confidence.

↶ **Here's the plan:** sit down, look over the exam, read all the directions, plan your approach, and schedule your time. If it works for me, then it should work for you.

♋ **Do the easiest questions first.** Getting those under your belt will give you confidence to go on to the harder ones.

♋ **Mark any questions** you don't know right off with some kind of symbol, and then go back to them later. Don't waste time getting stuck with any one question.

♋ **There have been times** in test situations where I really have felt overwhelmed by anxiety. I've learned that what I need to do at those times is to turn over my test, close my eyes, take three or four deep breaths, and grab hold of the situation before it gets totally out of control.

♋ **Whatever you do,** don't panic when other students start handing in their papers. Sometimes, those students are doing that because they've given up, not because they're better than you are!

♋ **When I finish a test,** I don't go over it with my friends. That just makes me more anxious. Instead, I reward myself. I buy myself something I wouldn't normally eat—like a big fat gooey cupcake—and I tell myself that, if nothing else, at least it's over for now.

♋ **One thing that I've come to understand** is that if I don't get a question, it may be because it's not a well-written test. You can do just as badly at creating a test as you can at taking it. So I'll ask the instructor. I've survived quite a few tests by doing that.

꧁ **Keep an eye out for clues** that are in the make-up of the questions themselves. For instance, if you're doing a True or False section, the words *always* or *never* usually indicate a false statement.

A lot of food for thought here on the subject of study skills. Now let's move on to skill-building in a whole other area: interpersonal relationships.

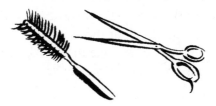

# Chapter 6

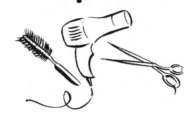

## WORKS AND PLAYS WELL WITH OTHERS

an you remember back to elementary school when you were graded on "Working and Playing Well with Others?" You could get an Excellent, a Good, a Satisfactory, or an Unsatisfactory. Well, guess what? Every day of our lives, we are *still* being graded on our skills in that area. The people around us—our teachers, our fellow students, our bosses and managers and coworkers, and our friends and family—are judging whether we are excellent, good, okay, or really not so hot at getting along with other people.

Part of what determines our aptitude for getting along with other people is the personality we project to the world. Some of us are blessed with sunny personalities that just naturally make people gravitate toward us. We are natural leaders who manage to convince others to do things our way; we are sought out and sought after, whether the context is professional or social. Others of us are quiet, reserved, or even seriously shy. Entering a group is a situation that we always feel we have to "rehearse" for. Our interactions are rarely spontaneous, but even so, they can still be successful and satisfying. Still others among us have significant problems fitting into a group altogether. We may be argumentative, hypercritical, sarcastic, suspicious, quick to pass judgment, ungenerous, even mean-spirited, or downright destructive.

Where do you see yourself fitting into any of the above descriptions? To answer that question, you have to look at yourself as objectively as you can, and maybe even solicit friends and family to help you make an assessment. It is only when you begin the work of self-assessment that you can start to make the changes that are necessary to help you function more effectively in group situations.

Personality is a complicated issue, but fortunately, we can all learn new and useful ways to interact with each other. In this chapter, you will be hearing from your fellow cosmetology students on ways that they have improved their interrelationships, with specific attention paid to such matters as communication, conflict resolution, and more.

# The Fundamentals of Communication

All relationships start with communication, though not necessarily spoken communication. An infant communicates with his or her mother at first in nonverbal ways. Two people sitting across from each other on a subway car can also communicate in non-verbal ways, particularly if the spark of an attraction is there. Communication is central to human existence, for if you cannot make your wants and needs known, or if you cannot hear others expressing their wants and needs, you're going to have a hard time being part of a team. And keep in mind that the ability to be a part of a team—to get along with your manager and your coworkers and your clients—will be a crucial factor in determining your ultimate success as a cosmetologist.

෴ **You know, when you think about it,** *everything* is communication. It's not just your words. The expression on your face, the way you make eye contact, and your body language all telegraph messages just as fast, if not faster, than words do. So if you want someone to get a message—or maybe even more important, if you don't want them to get a message—be aware of what your body language in saying. Folding your arms in front of your chest or slouching in your chair are statements that can be more powerful than a thousand words.

෴ **People from different cultures** communicate in different ways, and it's never too soon to start becoming aware of those differences. For example, in some cultures, if you look down at the floor when you're talking to someone, it's taken as a sign of respect. In other cultures, if you look down at the floor when you're talking to somebody, people are liable to think that you're shifty or that you've got something to hide.

⚲ **Do you ever run into people** who have absolutely no idea of what's an appropriate distance for two people to maintain when they're talking to each other? I hate that! It absolutely drives me crazy to have someone putting his face real close to mine and talking inches away from me. These people have obviously never heard about "personal space," and usually have no idea that they're invading yours. I once read somewhere how it's normal for family, lovers, and close friends to stand about a foot away from each other, but everyone else should keep four to 12 feet apart. Sometimes, I want to carry a sign around with me that says *Stay Behind the Line!*

⚲ **Pay attention** to the voice you use because your voice is going to have a huge impact on how effectively you communicate. If you're really loud or if you swallow your words, these are going to give people a message about who you are, and maybe the wrong message. Ask a friend to evaluate your voice. Does it need softening? Strengthening? Do you speak too fast or too slowly? Do a lot of people say, "Excuse me?" when you're talking to them?

⚲ **I have to admit** that I used to have this attention problem. I was fine as long as I was one on one with someone in a quiet place. But it you put me at a party or in any room where there was a lot going on, my attention would wander. I really alienated a few people

that way who thought I was always looking for someone more interesting to talk to. That really wasn't it at
all. I just have what's called "selective attention," and it
can be hard for me to focus in on one thing when
there are a lot of distractions going on around me.

---

## What Is Your Communication Style?

Just as different people can have different learning
styles, so different people can have different communication styles. Some of the more popular styles
include the following:

✄ *The Salesperson*   This communicator likes to
   touch and feel and talk. It's a very direct, open
   style, with little reluctance in approaching
   strangers.

✄ *The Thinker*   This communicator may be quite
   reserved, even guarded, but with excellent
   problem-solving abilities that will always make
   him a welcome member of a group.

✄ *The Relater*   This is the sort of person you can
   turn to and confide in, who interacts warmly,
   and genuinely seems to care about other
   people.

Of course, there are many other types. Look
around your classroom and see if you can name a
"type" for each of your fellow students, and for
yourself!

# Personality and Attitude

Right now, as a cosmetology student, you are dealing day to day with people. Once you are out there in the field, dealing with clients and fellow staff and management, your people skills will prove to be even more critical. It's probably safe to say that if you don't like to deal with people, another field might make more sense for you.

In assessing how you relate to people, it's helpful to make a distinction between personality and attitude. Someone can have an introverted personality and be shy, quiet, and reserved, but still have a positive attitude about other people. On the other hand, you might be an extroverted type—outgoing and always enjoying being at the center of attention—yet still have a fundamentally negative attitude about others. Attitude, on the other hand, is influenced or even formed by our environment: all the things we learn and take away from parents, teachers, peers, even books and movies. We may not be able to change a characteristic that we were born with, but we can certainly change our attitude.

 **Assertiveness was never a big part** of who I am. It just didn't factor into my attitude about life. I think a lot of women have trouble being assertive. I know my mother did, and my grandmother and all of my aunts and cousins. But once I got out into the world, where so many demands were being made on me and I realized I had to learn how to say no or I'd drown, I decided it was time to fine-tune my attitude and learn how to become more assertive. I did this with the help of books on the subject, and, finally, by going to a two-day workshop.

☙ **My soccer coach** in high school taught me the secret of assertiveness. He said it was a three-step process, with the key phrases being "I feel . . . I want . . . I will." For instance, I might say, "I *feel* I'm being taken advantage of in this situation." Then I step back and ask myself a few questions about what the situation really is. Then I might come up with something like, "I *want* to be valued as a person." Finally, get into the action mode: "I *will* make it clear that I do not allow myself to be treated disrespectfully." This method is a good, easy way to get into gear for dealing with tough situations.

☙ **My grandmother** was a real lady and she always said there was something we kids needed to learn: tact. "You don't have to say everything that comes into your head," she'd always tell us. "You can say it straight and be totally honest without being harsh or critical."

☙ **My sister** is a substance abuse counselor so she has a lot to say on the subject of attitude. She talks to her clients about "reframing." When you reframe, you adjust your attitude by essentially changing the meaning of an event. For instance, your teacher might say something to you like, "I think you can do better."

Now you might have a gut reaction to that where you're telling yourself that you've been put down and you're fuming. Reframing, however, gets you to put the brakes on those feelings. When you reframe, you might say something like, "My teacher's right. I could do better. And next time I will. Next time I'll really nail that assignment." Reframing slows you down so that you can turn any experience into an opportunity to learn.

✌ **Part of having a positive attitude** is being able to handle criticism. My father was always very critical of me, so criticism was something I saw as a very negative thing and I've had to work really hard to get better at accepting it. I used to withdraw or rationalize, and I can see, from my friends, that I wasn't alone in having a hard time handling criticism. Some of my friends try to blame other people whenever they're criticized. I've come to learn that the best way to handle criticism is to see it as a positive thing. It's feedback that can help you become better at what you do.

✌ **Too many people,** when they're criticized, rush to their own defense. I don't think that's such a great idea. If your teacher tells you you're not really focused, for instance, I don't think you should turn around and start telling her how you really are focused. I think it's better to say absolutely nothing and just listen. Later, after you've had a chance to reflect, then maybe you'll want to make a few points. But don't skip the reflecting part.

꙯ **When I get negative feedback,** I have to first consider who it's coming from. Do I respect this person? If the answer is yes, then I'll listen and I may ask for more specific information. Some people offer criticism in only general terms, and that doesn't help me very much. If I don't respect the person, then I won't pay any attention. That's just the way it is.

꙯ **I always go** for the "second opinion." For instance, if a teacher says to me, "You're disorganized," I'll take a survey of my friends and family. "Hey guys," I'll say. "Am I disorganized? Have you noticed this about me? Just how disorganized would you say I am?" It's a reality test, and even if it hurts, it's important to do.

꙯ **Giving negative feedback** can be as hard as getting it. In the future, when I'm part of a salon team, I'll probably be in the position where I'll have to give somebody some negative feedback at some point or another. The thing to remember is to criticize people only on those matters that you think they can change. If someone is clearly not a genius, it doesn't do any good to say, "You're not very smart." But things like organization and neatness and a sense of responsibility are qualities that almost all of us can improve on, to some degree or other.

꙯ **I've been an athlete** all my life. I lived and breathed basketball all through high school and junior high. I think being an athlete teaches some really basic skills about being part of a team. These skills come in handy when you're out in the real world. Like, one of the life lessons I've grown up with is the idea that you're not only concerned with your own success, but with the success of your teammates. When I'm doing a group project in school, I have a real sense that we've all got to pull together to make the project really work. I know that my sense of teamwork is going to be a strength for me in the years ahead.

☙ **Competition can be a healthy thing,** but only up to a point. It's a good external motivation, but it shouldn't get in the way of your relationships with people. If you're only thinking about yourself and being the best, then you're going to miss out on a lot of the special things you can get from other people.

☙ **I've got to laugh at people** who are so worried that you might learn something they know that you'll be a threat to them. We have this one girl in our class who's incredible at braiding, but if you ask her to show you anything, she runs off to the bathroom. You know what I mean? She reminds me of my Aunt Lillian, who made the world's best fried chicken but who'd never give the recipe to anyone. Well, Aunt Lillian died and that was the end of the world's best fried chicken. Some great memorial, huh?

# Conflict Resolution

Regardless of how positive your attitude is and how sunny your personality may be, you are bound to come into conflict with others along the way on the bumpy road of life. The way you handle and resolve conflict will have a lot to do with your ultimate success in school, in a job, and in life in general.

🕉 **Aim for neutrality.** There are going to be a lot of situations in life where people will try to pull you into a conflict and get you to "pick a side." Resist it. And resist the impulse to gossip. Like spitting out a car window, gossip will come back to hit you in the face.

🕉 **I try not to** take things so personally. Sometimes, people have a bad day and you just get hit by some flak. It doesn't have to be such a big deal all the time. Suck it up and move on.

🕉 **I used to be super-sensitive.** Now, as I get older, I've developed a tougher hide. If someone is brusque with me or gives me a funny look, I don't automatically assume that that person is out to get me. If I'm feeling really weird about how someone's acted toward me, I'll try to get that person alone in a quiet corner to ask her about it. A lot of times, I'll find out that it's a whole lot of nothing.

🕉 **Sure, there are "techniques"** to help you deal with conflict. But there are no real shortcuts. The foundation for healthy conflict resolution begins with you. When you fully understand who you are and what makes you tick, then you can begin to understand others.

🕉 **The best advice** I've ever been given on the subject of conflict resolution is that an ounce of prevention is worth a pound of cure. That means avoid getting into trouble in the first place and then you won't have to deal with the fallout. How do you avoid trouble? Well, to start with, don't get into the habit of gossiping about people. Loose lips sink ships and can make your life miserable if you've told somebody something about yourself or about someone else. As a student, if you gossip about another student, it's bad and it may come back to haunt you, but when you're a professional, out in the world, you've really got to understand that confidentiality is part of being a cosmetologist. You can't go around telling people that Mrs. Jones is bald or whatever. That's a sure way to end your career before it even starts.

☾ **If somebody says something** that I feel I have to disagree with, I always start with the word "I," not "You." This is something that I've learned as a parent. When my kid breaks a glass because he's been swinging a yo-yo in the kitchen, I don't start in by saying, "You're so bad! You're so clumsy! You never do anything right!" That's just chipping away at your kid's ego and it feels abusive to me. Instead, I put the action in the context of how I feel about it. I'll say something like, "I feel bad when you don't listen to me and accidents happen. I feel like I'm not able to make you hear me." That same approach is something you can learn to use with everyone in your life. Instead of telling a teacher, "You're going to fast," it's a lot better to say, "I'm having a hard time keeping up." Do you see the difference?

ɔ **Before you can hope to get good** at dealing with conflict, you've got to have an understanding of how anger works and the different ways that people deal with anger. Some people grow up in homes where it's against the law to be angry, so they turn their anger inside and become passive, only letting their aggression out in a lot of little ways. Other people are your "road-rage" types, going completely over the top with their anger. You need to be able to recognize "anger styles" and deal with them as they come up.

ɔ **I was taught** to turn the other cheek. Some people say that's not healthy—that you've got to get the anger out—but I don't know that I agree. Why should you get down to somebody else's level? You can be the big one.

ɔ **I'm not the kind of person** that gets involved in a lot of conflicts. I guess I'm just a pretty easygoing type. But whenever I do find myself in the middle of a dispute, I'll try to remember to use the other person's name. I'll say something like, "What's the problem, Matt?" or "What can we do to work this out, Leslie?" It shows that I see other people as people, even those individuals I may be having a conflict with, and it defuses their anger toward me.

ɔ **My grandfather always used to tell us** this thing that I carry with me to this day: "It is easy to make an enemy; it is harder to keep a friend." It's amazing how quickly a relationship can go bad and how hard it can be to fix a friendship after it's been damaged.

ॐ **When wolves get into a fight,** one of them makes itself submissive and shows its jugular to its enemy. This display usually puts a stop to the fighting. I learned from wolves. When I'm in a fight, I'll say something to the other person like, "You know, I really feel I could use your help to figure a way out of this mess." When I do this, the other person usually rushes to help me and I never feel like I've lost face. Quite the opposite. I feel like I've figured out a way to manage the situation like an adult.

ॐ **Laughing is a good response.** I don't mean in the other person's face, although sometimes it's hard to keep yourself from doing that. I mean finding somewhere in your day and life to have a good chuckle. If I'm having a problem, I'll go out for a drink with my friend Shelley, who is such a riot. She does these amazing impersonations of people in our class. After an hour with Shelley, I'm feeling no pain. She's like laughing gas for me.

ॐ **Listen, listen, listen.** Then listen some more. Some people, when they're in the middle of a conflict, are so anxious to state their case that they don't even hear what other people have to say.

ॐ **Never say or do anything** in haste and never, ever, write anything down! I think one of the worst inventions known to mankind is e-mail, in the sense that too many people, when they're angry, will go to their computer and jot off a furious note. Well, that e-mail becomes a historical record of your anger that you would rather not see again when you're feeling better. Use self-control in all your dealings and don't shoot off (or write off) at the mouth!

☾ **Before, after,** and, if possible, during a conflict, I'll try to share a good feeling with the other person. I'll figure out something good to say about her. That way, I can acknowledge that there's a problem but I put the problem in the context of something bigger. For example, I might say something like, "Jean, you always say what's on your mind and I admire you for that. But I'm not sure you understood me correctly blah blah blah." You see? It's a little dance. A give and take, which is a far cry from going in with both barrels and trying to blast a person to kingdom come.

☾ **Go for a walk** if you're feeling angry at someone. Breathe deeply. Eat a doughnut. Do something to break the chain of the anger. Then you can go back and look at the situation differently and decide the next best step.

☾ **In order to end the conflict,** it's important to ask yourself what you're looking for. For some people, it's an apology. The apology becomes like this pot of gold at the end of the rainbow. I try not to be so focused on apologies because some people will never apologize. It just goes against their grain and if you establish that as a condition, then you may never get over the anger. So instead of looking for apologies, I try to focus on coexistence.

☾ **When you're trying to iron out** a conflict with someone, always stay in the present. Always. Never bring up a whole history of who did what to whom. Once you start doing that, things will spiral out of control.

## Dealing with Teachers

Maybe you were intimidated by teachers or resentful of their authority at some point in your life. Don't let yourself get hung on such feelings now when you need to be as positive as you can to ensure your success. Here are some pointers from your fellow cosmetology students about ways to make sure your relationship with teachers is a good one:

✄ Make personal connections with your teachers, as it is natural to do so. Talk about your interests when you can. Maybe you'll find that your teacher also loves ballroom dancing or pottery or French films. That's a nice, easy way to connect.

✄ Participate as much as you can. It's hard work to teach to a class of stuffed owls. Teachers are very grateful to students who meet them halfway in terms of classroom discussion.

✄ Remember that teachers are people, too. They have good and bad days, just like everyone else. If they seem irritable, don't take it personally. Let it roll off of you.

# Dealing with Difficult People

You'd be surprised but it's possible to find yourself in a conflict with almost anyone, no matter how easygoing they may be. Things come up and anger cannot always be anticipated and avoided. Fortunately, however, most conflicts can be successfully resolved if both parties bring good will to the table. Chances are, however, that, in your years ahead, you will encounter downright difficult people, if you haven't done so already. When these difficult people turn out to be your coworkers, your bosses, or your clients, it can be a really tough situation. So let's have a heads-up on how we might deal with such people from some experienced cosmetologists who are out there in the field.

**I compliment these people.** Relentlessly. I have this one client . . . we'll call her Mrs. Jones. Mrs. Jones is the world's worst pain but I flatter her every inch of the way. "Mrs. Jones, don't you look lovely today." "Mrs. Jones, yellow is your color." "Oh, Mrs. Jones, you've got such a fascinating life." This may sound nauseating, but it's no skin off my back and it keeps everyone happy.

**One of my pals** in the salon had a huge blowout with another stylist, a woman I'll call Brenda. Now Brenda is a terrible troublemaker, a real spoiler kind of personality. My friend was fuming: she was going to tell Brenda off; she was going to go to the boss, yadda

yadda. I said, "Hold it right there. Send Brenda flowers instead." "What?" my friend cried. "You heard me." After we went back and forth a little, my friend did as I suggested and it worked like magic. At first, my friend thought that to send flowers would be an admission of guilt, but I told her that the more important thing was for her to look like a peacemaker in everyone else's eyes. That is exactly what happened.

 ℧ **When it comes to dealing with difficult people,** simply staying out of their line of view is the best strategy. It might sound really simple, but if you try using avoidance as a technique, you'll see how effective it is. I know in my salon we have one person who's a real problem, and you'd be surprised how many people, on their own steam, fly right into her orbit.

 ℧ **I think a little sympathy** and patience go a long way toward dealing with difficult people. Some of my friends call me "The Saint" because they know I have this attitude, but I'm comfortable with it. I feel that difficult people often have difficult lives or have had difficult childhoods, and I try to forgive them as much as I can.

 ℧ **Some of these people** are just plain bullies and you know what they say about bullies? If you stand up to them, they'll fold. I once had a manager who was riding me really hard so I got very direct with her. I said, "Gloria, you're harassing me. You're causing me psychological distress." Well, now, when you start using words like that, you can scare somebody pretty badly. Let me tell you, she clammed up fast.

As we said at the top of this chapter, the personal interactions we have with other people may very well determine whether we achieve real success or not in this field. Again, it is important to remember that the ability to get along with other people is a skill that can be learned, even if some of us are born more naturally with people skills than others. A vital part of the communication that is essential to good interrelationships is listening. Let us look at listening in more depth in the next chapter, where we will find out more about how to present ourselves to the world and how to project a good image.

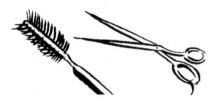

# Chapter 7

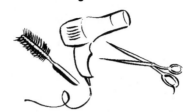

## WHAT DID YOU SAY?

f we had to name one skill that a cosmetologist absolutely has to master, that skill would be listening. Maybe you're great with your hands and can create cornrows better than anybody in the Western Hemisphere. Good for you. Maybe you're efficient beyond compare, always arriving at your job on time or early, and never screwing up appointments. Good for you. Maybe you have an incredible fashion sense and can tell just what color gown goes with what color hair, or what shape of haircut will enhance what shape face. Good for you. These talents are hugely important in the field of cosmetology and, if you can claim them, you'll be halfway to your goals for sure. But no matter how efficient you are or how good you are with your hands or your eyes, you may fall short of your ultimate goal if you cannot learn to listen.

Did you hear what we said?

Listening, unfortunately, is becoming a lost art in our society. In the centuries that came before the 20th century, people were taught the basics of communication. Young men and women courted each other in a formal fashion, and were taught how to carry on a conversation in a graceful way and how to present themselves to the world that would maximize their appeal. In modern times, these talents have taken a back seat to self-promotion, salesmanship, and other "skills" that are supposedly geared to helping you get along in a highly competitive society. As a cosmetologist-in-training, however, you have to learn the communication skills you may have neglected all these years while you were watching TV, walking around with headphones, or playing video games. You have to remind yourself that you have selected a service profession and, as such, a profession that comes with a set of rules you must follow. If you cannot learn to listen and to provide clients with what they want, then you will be making your work much harder than it has to be.

## Listen Up

Is good service really so much to ask for? Evidently, it must be, because poor service is regularly cited as one of the leading complaints about modern life.

Consider the following script, describing a customer putting in an order at a donut shop:

| Server: | May I help you, sir? |
| Customer: | I'd like a glazed donut, please. |
| Server: | How many donuts? |
| Customer: | One, please. |
| Server: | One powdered donut. |
| Customer: | Glazed, please. A glazed donut. |
| Server: | One powdered donut and one glazed donut. |
| Customer: | No! One powdered, I mean, glazed donut. And a cup of coffee with milk and two sugars. |
| Server: | One glazed donut and one cup of coffee with cream. |
| Customer: | Milk! |
| Server: | . . . with milk and one sugar. |
| Customer: | Two! |
| Server: | Two powdered donuts? |
| Customer: | One glazed donut! One cup of coffee with milk and two sugars. That's it! |
| Server: | Would you mind repeating that, sir? |

Sound familiar? Of course it does. Sound exasperating? You bet. Will you ever go into that donut shop again? Not if you're in a hurry and not if there's a better donut shop down the block. The same rule applies to the salon. If you're a stylist who doesn't know how to listen, your client will no doubt find a stylist who can, down the block at another salon.

Listening is the foundation of a good service relationship. But why is listening so hard? you ask. To this we reply, it doesn't have to be. Listening is a skill, like any other skill. If you practice it and work at it, you can learn to be a great listener with clients who appreciate how responsive you are. Let's "listen" to what your fellow cosmetology students have to say on the subject.

〰 **Communication involves a lot** of nonverbal cues. People usually nod their heads every now and then to show that they're listening.

〰 **Don't fall in love** with your own voice. Talk *to* people, not *at* them.

〰 **I practice listening** with my eyes closed. You'd be amazed how much more you hear.

〰 **To me, a big part of communication** has to do with asking good questions. It shows that you're curious and you're interested and you're there. I always keep question words in my head—Who? What? Where? When? Why? How?—and I use them a lot so I can get a better sense of what's going on.

〰 **Listening is part of the give and take** of communication. I know that, to some people, interrupting means you're not listening, but that's not necessarily the case. Interrupting is one of those cultural things that can mean one thing to one set of people and something altogether different to another set of people. Take my mom's family, for instance: they're all very quiet and polite. When someone is talking, no one would dream of uttering a word until that person is finished. Now in my dad's family, on the other hand, no one would ever dream of just sitting there like a bump on a log, waiting for the other person to finish. You interrupt! You get interrupted! You jump in whenever and wherever you can! Is it rude? It may look that way to the outside world, but there's nothing rude about it. That's just the way it is. It's another form of very active, engaged listening, that's all.

꠸ **One way to let people know** that you've been listening is to do this thing called "reflective listening." It's listening that reflects, or returns, the words to the speaker. If your teacher, for instance, says to you, "I like what you did in the front, but the back needs work," you might say, "I can see what you mean by the back needing work, but I'm glad to hear you like the front." This reflective listening reinforces what the other person has said so that the message sinks in.

꠸ **A good way to practice listening** is to use books-on-tape. I take out a books-on-tape from the library and I play them on the bus on the way to work so that I get myself in the habit of hearing.

# Client Communication

As a cosmetologist, it is very important that you learn to listen to your boss, to your manager, and to your fellow staff members. As we said in Chapter 6, you're part of a team, and you've got to demonstrate that you understand what that means. But bosses and managers and fellow staff members may be inclined to give you a second or a third or a fourth chance if you've been guilty of not listening to them. They get to see your skills on a day-to-day basis and they may choose to be forgiving about your listening lapses. Clients, however, may not be so tolerant. One strike and the game may be over. Chances are you've already been in the "lab" situation and have either been cutting a client's hair in your school setting or have assisted in some way. You are beginning to get a sense of how important client contact is. In this chapter, we are going to be focusing on ways to be with clients, with an emphasis, again, on listening.

## Meeting and Greeting

Never underestimate the importance of a first impression. You'd be surprised how hard you have to work to undo the damage of a negative first encounter. To safeguard against this, try some of the following tips. And remember: treat every visit as a first visit. It's a great way to stay out of trouble.

☙ **The job of a cosmetologist** is to make the client feel good. I always say that the best way to make someone feel good is to give him a nice big smile. It doesn't matter if your car is in the shop or your cat just had kittens or the pastrami sandwich you had for lunch isn't agreeing with you. The client is expecting a smile, so don't disappoint.

☙ **Our teachers always tell us** that the most important thing is to introduce yourself. If you don't use your name, how can you expect a client to make a connection with you, or when they're rebooking, to ask specifically for you?

꙳ **I always like it** when I go to a salon and somebody offers me coffee or some spring water. I'm going to do the same when the time comes.

# The Consultation

The consultation, which is the centerpiece of the stylist–client communication, has a very specific and focused purpose. The aim is to make sure that you and the client are on the same page regarding the service. As a student of cosmetology, you will soon begin practicing your consultation skills, so this is a good time for you to be hearing tips on the subject from those who are already out in the field.

꙳ **I know stylists** who skip the consultation altogether, or else only do it the first time they meet with a client. That's a big mistake, if you ask me. I factor consultation into every visit with every client, whether they like it or not.

꙳ **The consultation area** should be quiet enough for two people to be able to talk to each other, and it should be well equipped with style books, haircolor swatches, and a mannequin. And it has to be neat and clean: remember how important first impressions are. If the salon can't provide that, then you might want to look for a different salon.

꧁ **Make sure** your client is relaxed and comfortable when you begin the consultation. A cup of coffee does wonders.

꧁ **Keep your judgments to yourself** during the consultation. If the client says she colors, perms, or straightens her own hair, don't act like you've never heard of such a thing. The purpose of the consultation is to gather information. Later on, you can try to convince her to let you or someone else in the salon perform these services for her, but first you need to develop an atmosphere of communication and trust.

꧁ **A big part of the consultation** is getting a good hair history. You might have a style you're dying to try out on your client, but if you find out in the course of the consultation that the client has never spent more than five minutes a day tending to her hair and the style you're proposing requires a lot more maintenance than that, then you're just going to have to go back to the drawing board.

꧁ **Put the time in!** Don't rush the consultation process. People come in with set ideas in their heads, and if you want to "unset" them, you have to plan on having some extended conversation. For instance, the client may come in raving about some haircut that her friend got and you're going to have to take the time to guide her through the process, step by step, explaining why a cut that looks good on her friend might not look good on her.

C We've had some talented stylists in our salon who know how to give a great cut technically, but who have very little understanding of how a cut works with a client's total look. Part of the purpose of the consultation is to help you determine that total look. Does the client favor a classic look with tailored outfits and relatively conservative colors, or is she more drawn to whatever is trendy and hip? You also have to take into account the client's lifestyle. If she's a mom with two little kids under the age of five, don't suggest a style that's going to require any sort of real maintenance. It ain't gonna happen.

C It's important to understand the "dance" that goes on in the consultation. You have to lead. You have to take control of the situation. That means picking up on cues and clues from the client. You need to carefully watch her gestures and facial expressions during the conversation. Is she at ease or is she ill at ease? If she wants to go blonde, does she think it will make her look younger? Read her face and her body language when she answers. And don't forget reflective listening. Give her back what she gave you so you know whether you're both on the same page or not.

C Don't even think about doing a consultation without having a mirror handy. Even if it has to be a hand-held one, you're going to need it. When both of you look into the mirror together, you'll discover the things you see in common and the things you see differently.

☙ **One thing that is really important** to learn is never to promise the moon. If a client brings in a picture of some cover model and there's no way she's ever going to look like a cover model, don't pretend you're going to turn her into one. You can point out ways in which she can try to look like that model— the length of the hair, let's say—but in a tactful and discreet way, you're going to have to provide her with something of a reality test, too.

☙ **While you are going through** hairstyle books and discussing your client's particular needs, take this quiet moment to direct her attention to other services available at the salon. Let her know that in addition to a new haircut, she might also want to consider some of the salon's offerings in the areas of skin and nail care. Use the photos in the styling books to offer examples of these services. If you really want to succeed in this business, ticket upgrading has to always be in the back (or maybe even in the front) of your mind.

☙ **You may have a new client** who is unfamiliar with consultations. You'll want to let her know that it is salon policy to gather certain information before you can begin the service and so it is important for her to arrive early enough to fill out a consultation card. In many salons, the receptionist calls to remind clients about their appointment the day before it is scheduled. This is a good time to remind the client that she will need to fill out a consultation card, which will probably take her five to 10 minutes, with an additional 10 minutes or so for the two of you to talk it over.

# Consultation Cards

Don't even think about keeping the vital information you gather in a consultation just in your head. It will never stay there. You need records for everything you do.

**All service records** should include the name and address of the client, the date of each purchase or service, the amount charged, products used, and results obtained. Clients' preferences and tastes should also be noted.

**It's particularly vital for colorists** to keep accurate records detailing formulas, processing times, and any notes on porosity or other significant conditions. You might have a client who is absolutely thrilled with the magic you've worked on her hair and then, five weeks later, she's back for more and you have no idea what formula you used!

**Not only do I keep notes** of what I've actually done, but I write an ongoing narrative about how a service has turned out and what I think I could do better next time. I record my client's impressions and reservations, any goals I'm working toward, and so on. All of that goes down on the card.

**Make sure other people** can read your handwriting. If you happen to be out one day and a client needs to be serviced by another colorist, that colorist is going to have to read your notes.

〣 **There are good software programs** out there for storing and accessing all the color information and records you need.

〣 **My incredible discovery** for keeping records is a Palm Pilot. It stores many hundreds of records—believe me, I should have that many clients—and all I have to do is tap in whatever details I want and it all gets stored. The base color, the highlights . . . it's all there. My Palm also stores tons of other details about my clients like who referred them, their birthdays, what they do for a living, and so on. I love my Palm!

〣 **Once you've finished up** the service, you'll hear from the client whether she's satisfied or not. Take a few more minutes to record these results on the record card. Make a note of anything you did that you might want to do again, as well as anything that you wish you could undo, or at the very least, never re-peat. Also, make note of the condition of the client's hair after the service and jot down any retail products that you recommended for her purchase.

# Handling Client Problems

There's a law of nature that whatever can go wrong does go wrong. Some days, nothing could feel truer. You will have clients who arrive late and maybe you'll have dissatisfied clients. Here is some good advice on what to do in each of these cases.

## Tardy Clients

♋ **Clients who come late** can not only ruin your day but also can wreak havoc on the schedules of your other clients who may hold you responsible for their inconvenience. The first line of defense against tardy clients is for you to thoroughly familiarize yourself with the salon's lateness policy. I've found that the rule in most salons is that if a client is more than 15 minutes late, it's time to reschedule. I think that's really fair, don't you?

♋ **If your client freaks out** when you suggest rescheduling, don't you freak out, too. Calmly explain that you have other clients to take care of and you cannot rush them on account of another client's tardiness. If a client decides to take his business elsewhere as a result, so be it. That's the way the cookie crumbles.

♋ **If a client shows up late** and you can actually take him (let's say you had a cancellation in the following slot), don't let him off the hook right away. If you do, he'll probably be late again the next time. Try saying something like, "Lucky you! My next appointment isn't for another two hours, so even though you're twenty minutes late, I can take you." This telegraphs the message that lateness is not acceptable under normal circumstances, but in this case, you have decided to accommodate him.

♋ **Some clients** have this quirky thing about being late, but otherwise are perfectly fine people to deal with. I always schedule a client like that for the last appointment of the day.

↻ **Clients aren't the only ones** who run late, you know. It happens to everyone: me, too, sometimes. If I'm late, I'll call my clients to warn them in advance. I get all of my clients' phone numbers—at home, at work, or their mobiles—and I call them and give them the opportunity to reschedule. If I can't reach them, I'll go out to meet them when they arrive at the salon, apologize, get them coffee or mineral water, and maybe even slip in some free product at the end (even if it costs me out of my own pocket, it's worth it in the long run). That's usually enough to satisfy most people.

---

### Scheduling Mix-Ups

We all make mistakes. Here's how one stylist makes amends:

> If you get into a scheduling mix-up, don't make an argument out of whose fault it is. It just happened, that's all. The client is always right. You be the big one and assume all the blame. Believe me, you'll be glad you did. Just say, "I'm sorry. I messed up big time. Can I reschedule you?" Usually, when you throw yourself on somebody's mercy, they'll respond mercifully.

---

## Handling Unhappy Clients

There is no stylist who has not had the experience of having to deal with an unhappy, dissatisfied, and occasionally very vocal customer. It just comes with the territory. It helps, however, in dealing with the situation to remember that your goal is to make the client happy enough to pay for the service and to come back for more.

☙ **The first thing I do** is to try to find out why the client is so unhappy by asking specific questions. Not "Do you like it?" or "Don't you like it?" but what do you like? For example, "Are you happy with the length of the bangs?" "Does the length at the nape of the neck work for you?" "Would you like me to take off more around the ears?" It's a game of hot and cold. Your questions should let you know when and if you get warm.

☙ **If the customer wants** something changed and you can change it, then go for it! For instance, if she hates the color, look at your book and check the earliest time that you can schedule an appointment to undo what you've done. If you're full up, you'll have to explain to her that you will need to enlist the help of another stylist to fix what she's unhappy with. This isn't going to be music to her ears, but she'll have to understand that this is the way it's done.

☙ **Sometimes what is done** cannot be undone. This is a hard truth about life. If you've cut the hair too short, you can't make it grow back. If this is the case, you'll just have to take the bull by the horns, admit the truth, offer any options that might help the matter like conditioning treatments or other styling options, and let the chips fall where they may. Maybe your honesty will help unruffle the client's ruffled feathers or maybe she'll never come back again. You'll find out.

✺ **I used to work next to this guy** who, when he had an unhappy client, would just keep telling her how great she looked. "Are you crazy? It's fabulous on you! Fabulous!" Guess how many unhappy clients he managed to convince?

✺ **Okay, here comes the nightmare.** You're young, you're inexperienced, and you've messed up big time. Maybe you've cut all wrong around the ears; maybe your color came out orange and you haven't a clue what to do. Don't tough it out. Go to a more experienced stylist or to your manager for help. This can be done quietly; the client never has to know.

✺ **Sometimes you just can't win.** Your client is unhappy and nothing you say can calm him down. Maybe he's not such an easy person to start with. This is the time to seek help from your manager. It won't reflect poorly on you; helping out in these situations is a manager's job.

✺ **Try to schedule a few minutes** with your manager after you've been through an experience with an unhappy client. If the manager is any good at managing, you won't walk away feeling worse. It will be a growth opportunity and a good chance to examine the experience from all angles.

〜 **Our salon has a** "three times, you're out" policy. In other words, if a client complains three times about the same person or three times about three different people, we say "Bye-Bye." Life is too short. Three attempts to please a person are all we can afford. Keep in mind that there are some people who can never be pleased, no matter how hard you try.

〜 **We regularly do client surveys** in our salon. We offer the clients a 20 percent coupon on retail if the person fills out a survey. You can learn a lot about keeping customers happy from a good survey.

All of the tips you've just read will prove useful in helping you achieve satisfying communications with your clients. In the chapter that follows, however, we will be returning to the things you have to do for yourself in order to ensure your success in this field.

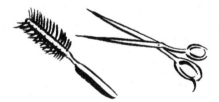

# Chapter 8

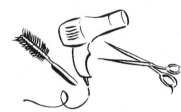

## HOLISTIC HINTS

**W**e don't have to tell you that a student's life is a hard one. You're working overtime to master the information you need to know, and chances are you're doing it while you're working part time or more in a job. Throw in a kid or two or three, as is the case with so many of you, and the overload can really get crazy. Living the life of a cosmetology student can be a little bit like running a marathon and jumping hurdles at the same time, and you wouldn't try that without getting yourself into good shape physically, would you?

The overload doesn't necessarily stop when you get out of school either. As a working cosmetologist, the pressure is often turned up to high. If business is good, you can expect to be heavily booked. Countless demands will be made on you and there is always the stressful potential for making mistakes. The need to keep yourself in good mental and physical condition will continue throughout your career. Starting now, you have to get into the habit of looking at "The Whole You."

The idea of "wholeness" is at the heart of the word *holistic*, which means "to emphasize the organic or functional relation between the parts and the whole of something." If we take a "holistic approach" to our lives, we are seeing ourselves as whole people.

In adopting a holistic approach to life, we take into account the mind, the body, and the spirit, and we examine how they interact and impact on each other. To neglect one will, over time, negatively affect another. In this chapter, we will be looking at ways to hold all the parts of ourselves together in order to stay healthy and whole.

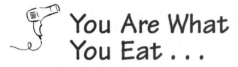

# You Are What You Eat . . .

. . . is a famous old saying, and as is the case with many famous old sayings, there's a lot of truth to it. What we put into our bodies has a great deal of bearing on how well we can expect to function. Let's hear what your colleagues in the field have to say on the subject of nutrition.

❧ **What's the single most important piece** of nutritional advice you'll ever hear? Drink water! It is so crucial to keep yourself hydrated. Sixty percent to seventy percent of our bodies are water, so if you think of how much we lose during the day, sweating and going to the bathroom and what have you, you'll realize how important it is to replace those fluids. The more you drink, the better you'll feel and function. I try to drink at least eight glasses of water a day. I won't go anywhere without my water. I always keep it with me and I drink *before* I get thirsty.

✣ **If you're looking to make smart choices,** drink water and mostly water. Other liquids, like tea and coffee, can act as diuretics, actually causing water to leave your body. Also, why do you need the calories in colas or the chemicals in diet colas or the expense of drinking fancy juices or bottled shakes when water is so cheap, so healthy, so nonfattening, and so refreshing?

✣ **I agree** with what the others have to say about the importance of water, but like everything else, you don't want to overdo. I've heard of people who were drinking gallons of water a day, and that can be dangerous, too.

✣ **Like most people** in the world, I've been on every kind of cockamamie diet. Grapefruit, cabbage soup, some diet where I was eating steak five times a week and almost went broke. Now I just eat with variety and moderation. I'll eat grains, fruits, veggies, a little chicken or fish, a little dairy. I cover my bases.

✣ **My little Italian grandmother** is so healthy. She's 89 now and still pours olive oil over everything she eats. But she's also eating fruits and vegetables, and the way she eats meat is like a tiny serving once a week, like a garnish on her plate. She's going to live forever, that one.

〰 **When it comes to food,** it's not just the food group or the amount that's important. It's the quality of the food. I always make a point of eating whole foods. Slow foods, they're calling it these days, as compared to fast food. I'm talking about foods that have the least processing. Real cheese instead of cheese food. Rolled oats instead of some sugar-packed cereal. Even a piece of semisweet chocolate if I have a sugar craving over some candy bar that's stuffed with marshmallow-nougat-brittle and that may have all kinds of artificial ingredients in it. When it comes to food, the less you mess with it, the better.

〰 **I had this sign made up,** all laminated and everything, and I stuck it on my fridge. It says, Do not eat when you're not hungry. Most of the time you're doing that, you're just trying to make up for stress, which can be better dealt with anyway by a few minutes of deep breathing or a walk in the fresh air. You'd be amazed how much easier it is to keep your weight under control when you pay attention to your stomach hunger instead of your mouth hunger.

〰 **My mothe**r always used to tell me to chew each bite of food 50 times. She drove me crazy, but you know what? Now I can see there's a lot of sense to it. As an adult, I find that if I eat slowly and chew my food thoroughly, I eat a lot less and my stomach is a lot happier.

�™ **Watch your portions.** Americans are known throughout the world for eating totally excessive amounts of food. The idea of "doubling" it or ordering a 64-ounce soda is unheard of in most parts of the globe and should be unheard of here, too.

☙ **I always bring my lunch** from home. Even if I'm going out with a friend, I'd rather brown bag it with some good healthy food than wind up eating in some overpriced restaurant where the food isn't even that good. And don't even get me started on fast food! Some of the students here go out for lunch to those places every day and I just want to say, "Do you see what you're putting in your body, honey? Can't you do better than that? Don't you have a kitchen at home?"

☙ **Suddenly,** "fat" has become a dirty word. That's ridiculous. There are good fats and bad fats. The good fats, like those we get from olive oil and nuts and stuff are really, really good for you. The bad fats, like animal fats and tropical oils, are bad for you. Good fats are delicious and satisfying and a little bit will satisfy your hunger. When we cut down on fat, we bulk up on carbohydrates, which, for most people mean highly refined foods like sugar, pastas, and white breads. Or maybe you'll start stuffing "lite" foods, thinking that they can't hurt you. Ha! Just watch the scale.

❧ **Don't worry so much** about your protein intake. You don't have to eat meat, fish, or chicken for protein. Think about beans and nuts, tofu, or maybe a protein supplement added to a smoothie or a shake. That's what I do. Every day I put a full measure of protein powder in a blender with some O.J. and a frozen banana and I don't have to worry about my daily protein intake at all.

❧ **I've got a secret** to eating healthy: make every meal a nice meal. If you take time with your food and think about the overall experience of eating, you'll be a lot less likely to stuff your face. For breakfast, I always make sure there's some beautiful fruit on the plate. For lunch I like hot soup in a thermos. When it's time for dinner, even if I'm home alone, I'll put down a placemat, pour myself a glass of wine, and eat a leisurely and relaxing meal. Taking care of myself that way really recharges me.

❧ **I just want to say a word** on behalf of fiber. You've got to make sure you have it in your diet. That means fruits, vegetables, legumes, whole-grain breads, and cereals. Better do it now, folks, or you'll be paying for it later.

❧ **Short of a banana** or an apple, I don't eat anything unless I read the label first. I want to find out how much fat is in it, what kind of fat, how much sodium, if there are any calcium benefits, and so on. My family thinks I'm nuts but I don't care.

# Getting Fit . . . Staying Fit

Factoring exercise into an already busy life isn't easy, but some form of regular exercise is vital if you want to keep your body, mind, and spirit in working order. Obviously, in our fitness-obsessed culture, there are reams to read about what makes for a good exercise program. We've culled your fellow cosmetology students for a "Top Ten" of helpful hints.

☾ **Hey,** you're not in this for the Olympics, are you? You're just trying to get something good going for yourself. Something good generally means something in the neighborhood of three to five exercise sessions a week, anywhere from a half hour to an hour per session. Now doesn't that sound doable?

☾ **Lots of people** hate exercise because they think it's boring. Well, the truth is it is kind of boring, at least until the exercise high kicks in, which in most cases, doesn't happen until you find your groove. I think the ticket is to pick a repetitive motion that you don't mind so much. For some people, that means walking; for others, running. Some of us like to swim while some people prefer to ride a bike (or a bicycle machine). It's your choice. Just choose something.

☾ **My vote** goes to dancing. If you can let yourself get into it, you'll probably have more fun exercising that way than any other way you can think of. Take a dancercise class or if you really want to try something awesome, find some square dancing somewhere.

☙ **I always look for ways** that I can up my exercise output. Like I'll take two steps at a time when I'm walking up a staircase or better yet, I'll walk the whole way instead of taking an elevator. When I go to the mall, instead of circling for twenty minutes looking for a parking spot that's close to the stores, I'll park really far away and walk twenty minutes.

☙ **Get yourself an exercise buddy.** Having somebody to share the fun and the agonies with is worth a lot.

☙ **I know that if I really want exercise** to be a part of my life, I have to do it the same time of day so I know I'm not going to be interrupted.

☙ **There's an expression** I've heard: train, don't strain. If you're hurting or if you're breathing too hard to be able to carry on a conversation, you may be doing something wrong. To make sure you're doing what you should be doing, check with your physician before starting any kind of exercise program.

☙ **I like to track my progress.** I keep a chart of what I've done from day to day, week to week, month to month. When I'm feeling burned out on exercise, this display of how far I've come inspires me to go further.

☙ **Interval training** has been really effective for me. That means I run two minutes really fast, then two minutes slow, then two minutes fast, then two minutes slow. Feels good.

꙾ **Breathe deeply,** several times a day. A lot of us run around too busy to take a deep breath. Deep breathing aerates your lungs and makes you better able to do the exercise you set out to do.

# Physical Presentation

A major part of how you can protect your physical self is to make sure that you handle your "physical presentation" in a healthy and solid way. To a large degree, your physical presentation is made up of your posture, your walk, and other movements. Your physical presentation can either enhance your attractiveness or take away from it, but it is also an important factor in determining your overall well-being. Unhealthy or defective body postures can cause a number of musculoskeletal problems, particularly when these postures become habit. Here are some ideas from your colleagues about how to keep your body in good shape while working in a salon environment:

꙾ **My aunt,** who's been a cosmetologist forever, has given me a lot of great tips about posture. She's got this set of rules you have to live by and it goes like this: Head up and chin level with the floor; neck stretched and balanced directly above the shoulders; chest out and up; shoulders level; spine straight; abdomen flat; hips level horizontally; knees slightly flexed and positioned over the feet. At first, when you do this, you feel like it's impossible, but once you've got it down, it keeps you in good shape for your entire career, according to my aunt.

↺ **Sitting is not something** people usually give a lot of thought to, but when you're sitting all day—like if you're doing nail care, let's say—you'd better believe that there's a right way to sit and a wrong way to sit. The right way is to slide your rear to the rear of the chair. This may not feel that natural at first, particularly if you sprawl in your chair like I do. But you'll see: if you tuck your fanny into the back of the chair, your body will be a lot happier at the end of the day.

↺ **I was sitting on a stool** in class one day and the teacher said to me, "It's designed for your entire bottom, dear." She was right. I was only halfway on, and when I really planted myself on the stool, it felt a lot better.

↺ **When you're sitting,** keep your back straight and the soles of your feet on the floor. Don't cross your legs or your feet at the ankle. Your soles on the floor help give you support.

↺ **You know what my teacher says** is the absolute worst thing a stylist can do? Work in high heels. It doesn't matter if the heels are chunky or narrow. Either way, you're putting pressure on your knees and throwing off your center of gravity, which leaves you open to back pain and arthritis. High heels are for weddings: your wedding!

ᔕ **Get yourself a good pair of shoes.** No, get yourself at least two good pairs of shoes. Something nice and wide and low-heeled that will absorb shock and give your toes the room they need. Don't leave home without them!

ᔕ **When you get yourself a job** in a salon, if it's not carpeted, you should treat yourself to a cushioned mat for your station. It'll go a long way toward beating fatigue.

ᔕ **All of us working in this field** are very susceptible to CTDs. That's cumulative trauma disorders, in case you didn't know. We have to stand all day and hold our bodies in unnatural positions for long periods of time, which means we're contracting our muscles. This can lead to problems of the hands, wrists, shoulders, neck, back, feet, and legs. Prevention is the key here. We've got to fit the work to our bodies, not our bodies to the work.

ᔕ **There are certain ergonomic measures** we all have to be aware of. One of them is to adjust the height of your chair with each client, and to swivel the chair as much as you need to so you're not overextending your reach.

ᔕ **People lapse into bad habits,** even those of us with good technique. So what I do is I have another stylist watch me now and then to make sure I'm not doing anything I shouldn't be doing. I ask them to evaluate my technique, and maybe they'll tell me that I'm not keeping my wrists as straight as I should or whatever, and so I'll make corrections.

ℭ **I always hold** my blow-dryer sideways. That way, I don't raise my arms above shoulder level any more than I have to.

ℭ **Sharp shears** make a big difference. If your shears are sharp, well balanced, and well lubricated, you won't have to work so hard when you're cutting hair.

ℭ **Keep your elbows** as close to your sides as possible.

ℭ **I always try** to keep my back straight and I always, always, always bend at the hips or knees instead of at the waist.

ℭ **Study the flamingo:** they stand for long periods of time by resting on one foot. If you're standing for a long time, try placing one foot on a stool for a while. You'll see the difference.

ℭ **When you're giving a manicure,** always have your client extend her hand across the table to you, not the other way around. If you're extending your hands and arms all day to your clients, you'll wear yourself out in no time.

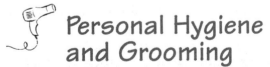

# Personal Hygiene and Grooming

As you train to become a cosmetologist, it is important for you to always keep in mind that you are in the image business. People will be coming to you so that you can make them look good. If you don't look good yourself, your clients may worry that you can't make them look good. Looking good always starts with good personal hygiene. Most of the issues around personal hygiene are obvious and we will not insult your intelligence by even bringing them up here. Surely you understand the importance of tooth-brushes and deodorants. Your grooming is also going to be looked at carefully. Here are some helpful hints from cosmetologists already out in the field that you should think about incorporating into your lifestyle.

☾ **The three most important words** in your life? Wash your hands! Making this simple and free practice a religion will save you and your clients an enormous amount of grief.

☾ **It seems as if** I shouldn't have to tell other cosmetologists about the need to moisturize, but it's too important a hygiene issue to go unmentioned. Skin dries out so quickly, especially under conditions like central heating or air-conditioning, exposure to the sun, and what have you. Find a moisturizer you like and live with it. Carry it with you everywhere. Use it on your face and your hands throughout the day. An ounce of prevention is worth pounds of cure!

☾ **Everything about you** is going to be an advertisement to your clients. That means your hair and certainly your nails. Ragged, dirty nails will turn off clients. Why should they place their trust in someone who can't live up to the standard they're aiming for?

✍ **We cosmetologists** are in a people profession. We get very close to others throughout the day. To me, that means no garlic on the pizza. Seriously. I mean, I love garlic on pizza but I'm not going to lose a client on account of it. And believe me, you do lose clients over things like bad breath.

✍ **Lose the perfume.** A great many people are allergic to fragrances, and more and more salons are instituting a no-fragrance policy. If you feel you absolutely have to use fragrance, keep it as light as you can. A citrusy toilet water, for instance; never some heavy, musky scent.

✍ **I am personally quite surprised** and sometimes appalled by the way some of my coworkers, particularly the younger ones, maintain—or should I say, fail to maintain—their wardrobes. Clothing is stained or ripped. Buttons are missing. Sweaters are so pilled as to be unsightly. Whites are yellowed. Don't they understand the first thing about what you need to do to keep yourself looking fresh?

✍ **My pet peeve** is crummy looking shoes. Some people will really put themselves together and look just fine until you get down to their feet. Shoes need to be cleaned, like any other part of your wardrobe, and a good polish helps, too. Downtrodden heels aren't the world's best look either. I know it's hard to find a shoemaker these days, but that doesn't mean that you can get away with shoes that look like junk.

✌ **Fact of life:** some people's feet don't smell so good. That's probably because they perspire a lot, which is healthy and fine and is usually addressed by civilized people with underarm deodorant. But people perspire through the soles of their feet as well, you know, particularly when you're on your feet all day long walking the equivalent of I don't know how many miles. So I always keep a natural foot powder on hand and I use it liberally during the day.

✌ **I try to kindly and gently suggest** to some of the youngsters who come to work here that they don't have to show up looking like Christmas trees. You know what I mean? Some of them wear so much jewelry and try for so much flash. It's a lot to keep up and can be very distracting. As a manager, I would tell a young stylist that it's a good idea to try to have her hair, makeup, and clothing blend in with the surroundings of the salon. Look around the salon. If everyone is very minimalist, don't come in looking like the Queen of Diamonds. It's only common sense.

✌ **As a manager,** I think there's a lot to be said for uniforms. I love working in a salon where everyone is wearing the same crisp, clean, and smartly-cut outfit. It feels very professional and easy to me.

✌ **Uniforms can be a great solution** for the salon, but even if you're working in a salon with a "no-uniform" policy, you might want to create a "uniform" of your own. In other words, keep your wardrobe very simple, classic, and easy, and you'll convey a sense of style and utility that others will want to copy. I think good choices for such a "uniform" are simple A-line skirts in muted colors with a white or black silk T-shirt, for instance. For a guy, it might be a white shirt, a tie, and clean, tailored khakis. These "uniforms" project just the kind of professional appearance and attitude that may allow you to charge more for your services.

☽ **It's one of those weird quirks** of human nature, but did you ever notice how someone who's a builder can have the most run-down home? I've known hairdressers like that. They cut other people's hair all day long and they allow their own hair to get long and ratty or faded. Bad idea!

☽ **One little (well, maybe not so little) thing** that drives me crazy: I see some of the other girls in the salon sharing makeup. That is such a bad idea! Makeup is a breeding ground for bacteria and should never be shared with anyone else. Sharing can lead to conjunctivitis, sties, herpes, and don't ask! I keep makeup for six months and then I get rid of it. I start in with new, fresh makeup that's just for me.

We've covered quite a bit of material in this chapter about how to keep yourself in good physical condition and how to present yourself to the world in a way that makes you look good while you're feeling good. There is one area, however, that has to do with your physical self that is so important we are devoting a whole chapter to it. That is the area of stress, coming right up.

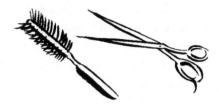

# Chapter 9

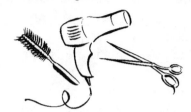

## I CAN'T HANDLE THIS!

eadaches. Poor sleeping. Overeating or undereating. Lack of sexual interest. Little enjoyment in day-to-day life.

Is any of the above striking close to home? If so, you may be suffering from too much stress.

What is stress? It can be defined as an environmental condition that causes physiological changes (those that have to do with our bodies), cognitive changes (those that alter the way we think), emotional changes, and behavioral changes. For instance, let's imagine that you are about to take your licensure exam. As you sit down and set out your pencils and your bottled water, you realize that you are in an environmental condition that is causing you big-time stress. The physiological changes are there: your palms are sweaty, your hands are cold, your heart is pounding, and your head aches. Emotional changes may be present: you could be feeling panic, despair, or who knows what. Behavioral changes? Maybe you're giddy, and much to the annoyance of those around you, you are chattering your head off. Cognitive changes? Perhaps you are so stressed out that you can't even think straight and are unable to focus in on the exam.

Stress, as you know, is often a counterproductive, self-defeating thing. Too much of it can be a killer. Stress can impact in very serious ways on your body and is a huge concern for people in the world today. In fact, there's so much of it in our modern world that the World Health Organization has designated it as an epidemic.

Stress is very prevalent in the field of cosmetology where you must perform at a high level with clients and staff. Mistakes are made, of course, but too many mistakes may result in your reputation being reconsidered. When you put all the physical demands of the job on top of that kind of pressure, you can wind up with a heavy load of stress.

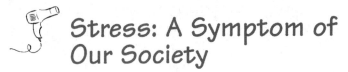 ## Stress: A Symptom of Our Society

Before we get into the specific kinds of stress that cosmetologists are subject to, let's spend a few moments thinking about the role that stress plays in the lives of us all. We live in a stressful world. To start with, many of us are seriously sleep-deprived. Americans don't get nearly enough vacation time compared with workers in Europe who routinely get two whole months of paid vacation a year, as well as generous maternity and paternity leaves. In the United States, in spite of our great national wealth, issues like child care and health insurance can become sources of major stress for our citizens. The stress picture doesn't get any better when we, as commuters, find ourselves on congested thoroughfares trying to get to our jobs on time. Consider, too, periods of economic downturn, and you can see that we have a very stressed population indeed. And all of the above is routine, everyday stress, which doesn't take into account the major stressors that occur in people's lives like the deaths of loved ones, illness, divorce, economic reversals, and so on. So how are people like yourself dealing with that kind of stress? Let's hear what your colleagues in the field have to say on the subject of stress: how to recognize it, how to handle it, and how to beat it.

**♋ Half the time,** I might not even know how stressed out I am until somebody points it out to me. "You're not eating" or "Look how fast you're eating" or "Why are you grinding your teeth?" Then I'll stop and think about what I'm doing and, sure enough, I'm stressed to the max.

**♋ When I'm stressed,** all the energy drains out of me. All I want to do is sleep. And so that's what I wind up doing. I go home, I eat cereal for dinner, and I go to sleep.

♋ **I get really compulsive** when I'm stressed. I eat tons and tons of chocolate. Fortunately, I'm one of those people who never gains weight so it doesn't show on me, but how healthy can it be? Still, it's better than what my girlfriend does. When she's stressed, she goes out shopping. You ought to see her bills.

♋ **Hey, it's not the end of the world** to have some stress in your life. These days, the media tell us that if we have stress we're going to keel over. Do you think there has ever been a time in human history when people didn't feel stress like when they were burning people at the stake and marching off to war? Do you think that was any bed of roses? You've got to tough yourself up a little.

♋ **I think in a lot of ways** we're a soft society. My grandparents had a lot of stress in their lives. They lived through the Depression and World War II but they were doers. Today, a lot of people just fold over if they have stress or else they run out and get the latest recreational drug. If you ask me, a little stress can be an energizing thing. I like the stress I feel, for instance, when I go in to take an exam. It takes me up a few notches so that I perform at my best.

♋ **I always thought I was basically okay** at handling stress and then all of this happened. Oh boy. I lost my job and spent three months before I found another salon I could feel comfortable in. My boyfriend and I split up. My mom got a virus that turned into endocarditis and had to spend two weeks in the hospital. I tried all the meditation and exercise stuff that usually works to keep my stress under control, but it wasn't working. So for now, I'm taking an anti-anxiety drug. I'm not going to be on it forever, but it's really helped me get through the bad stuff.

↻ **I think you've got to acknowledge** the difference between "stress" and "distress." Stress is what hits you on a day-to-day level if you're in a high-pressure job. You cope with it, just like you cope with your mother-in-law if she's a problem or that construction that's been tying up your commute for the last six months. Distress is what you get when you feel like you can't get away from the stress. That's when the headaches kick in and the acid reflux and that whole bit.

---

### Recognizing Signs of Stress

Stress impacts us in a wide variety of ways:

*Physical*   digestive problems, headache, neck pain, skin rashes, muscle tension, elevated blood pressure, flare-ups of illnesses like arthritis or asthma

*Thought processes*   memory issues, impatience, procrastination, obsessive behavior

*Emotional*   depression, irritability, helplessness, anxiety, anger, bitterness, conflicts with coworkers

If you are chronically suffering from these sorts of symptoms, consult with your physician to determine the best course of action.

---

# Stress and the Cosmetology Student

As we said above, all of us in this modern world are subject to stress. But you, as a cosmetology student, have a whole other level of things to feel stressed about. How you handle that stress will determine how likely you are to achieve your ultimate goals.

☙ **Sometimes, I can't believe** I'm a student again. I mean, I was never exactly a shining star in high school. Sometimes I feel completely overwhelmed. How am I going to get through this? How am I going to learn everything I need to know?

☙ **I just, like, glaze over** when I have to read some of that stuff in the textbook. Like things about chemistry and electricity, stuff like alkanolamines and iontophoresis. Give me a break! I get so stressed when I see that stuff that I feel like the top of my head's going to shear off. And when I have to get tested on all of that, my mouth goes so dry I can't even talk.

☙ **You want to know what makes me crazy?** It's the money. I was working at a salon before I went to cosmetology school and I was doing really nicely, thank you very much. I had money for restaurants, concerts, even a trip to Florida. Then I decided to go to school so I could get my license, and suddenly I'm working for half of what I was and I've got tuition to pay and when the bills come on the first of the month I get so stressed that my kids know not to come near me. "Mommy's got bills," they say. Boy, does Mommy have bills!

⟳ **Sometimes, I'll just feel totally stressed** about whether I've made the right decision. Even just saying that out loud stresses me out so bad. But how do I know? I've made mistakes before. I was going to be a travel agent and then I worked the front desk of a hotel for a while, and with those two experiences, I didn't exactly hit the ball out of the park, if you know what I mean. So now I feel like I'm on my third-choice career and how do I know I'll be any better at this one? It scares the life out of me sometimes.

⟳ **I'm totally freaked out** about the licensing exam. I don't do well with tests in general—I never have—so the idea of going into one that's going to have so much impact on my present and my future is really heavy. Like, I don't know if I can do pin curls the way you're supposed to. I don't know if I'll ever be able to do pin curls the way you're supposed to!

⟳ **Why is this field so stressful?** Because you have to perform for clients as well as for your boss. You have to be technically excellent and you have to be able to get along with people. You have to be able to organize your time and you have to be able to sell stuff, which for some people is one of the most stressful aspects of the field. Throw into all this the fact that you are dealing with an incredibly wide and unpredictable range of personalities and the fact that you're on your feet all day. And what do you get? Stress!

**I've become very aware** over the years that whatever stress I'm having at home, I'm going to wind up bringing into the salon with me. Whether it's with my husband or my kids or my mother or my kid's principal, it's going to find its way into the salon. Just knowing that makes me better able to control things. There's also stress from factors that have nothing to do with people. I might be having a bad reaction to some substance I'm using at work, for instance, and this could be causing me and my body a load of stress.

# Stress Relief: The Big Picture

Relief from stress comes in two ways: by changing or modifying your behavior and by adopting whatever methods help you to control the stress you experience. Let's start by looking at the behavior modification that may be necessary.

## Assertiveness

One of the most significant "big picture" sources of stress has to do with the issue of assertiveness. Are you the kind of person who always feels that you're being forced into doing something you don't want to do? Do you have a hard time expressing your feelings and saying no? If so, you are probably feeling put upon a great deal of the time, and this may be causing you great stress. Fortunately, there are proven methods to help you become a more assertive person who feels more on top of things.

What exactly is assertiveness? Let's think of it as the ability to express yourself and to verbalize your rights without violating another person's rights. It is the opposite of road rage, wherein your expression takes a completely aggressive and destructive form. An assertive person expresses thoughts and feelings in a way that clearly states the underlying needs. A person who is successful at becoming positively assertive is also able to keep open the lines of communication with others.

To become assertive—and again, we want you to think of this as a positive word—you should have a firm understanding of your rights as a human being. The U.S. Constitution is founded on the belief that all Americans have the rights of life, liberty, and the pursuit of happiness. Your personal "constitution" should include those same three, of course, but you should also understand that you have the right to decide on how to live your life. Your goals and dreams should be your own. You have the right to claim your own values, beliefs, and opinions. If you choose to believe in an all-powerful entity or not is your right. If you wish to believe in the institution of marriage or if you decide that marriage is not relevant to you is your right. You have the right as well to express yourself. That means saying "No" or "I don't understand" or whatever else you wish to say. You have the right to ask for information and help as you need it. You have the right to make mistakes and to fail at something, as long as you understand that it is you who will be dealing with the after-effects of your decisions.

Assertiveness is different—very different—from selfishness. Selfishness rides over the rights of other people. Assertiveness expresses your own rights with the understanding that individuals must coexist. Assertiveness is no magic bullet. It will not cure you of all your problems, but it will allow you to say "no" or "yes" as the situation arises. And for many people, learning how to say "no" or "yes" is half the battle.

Let's look at some ways that your fellow students have learned how to make assertiveness a part of their lives.

✧ **I've learned to live by** two small words: *be clear.* Let people know what's on your mind and let them know in a way that is to the point and on target.

✧ **I practice** using certain key phrases. "I want to" or "I don't want to." "I disagree" is another one. "I have a mixed reaction to what you're saying." These are the kinds of expressions by which you make yourself clear without any display of anger.

✧ **Assertiveness comes more easily,** and more effectively, when you have one-on-one exchanges with people. If you have a problem with something that someone has done, don't tell the person through someone else or when you're in a group situation with that person. Take it into a private corner somewhere.

♋ **One of the rules of assertiveness** is to own the feeling you're having. That means if you have a problem with something, put it in personal terms. "I don't agree with what you said," is a far better thing to say to somebody than "you're wrong," which leaves no room to go anywhere. "I'd like you to pick up the dry cleaning" is a better thing to say to your husband than "you have to pick up the dry cleaning." Hear the difference?

♋ **Part of getting good** at assertiveness has to do with allowing for feedback. Keep in mind that assertiveness doesn't mean it's all about you. The point of assertiveness is to keep the lines of communication open. Saying things like "Am I making myself clear?" or "What are your feelings about this?" are ways to be assertive and yet to still make it clear that you're looking for a dialogue.

---

### Learning to Say "No"

Learning to say "no" is the hardest thing in the world for some people. You've got to practice it, because if you don't get it down, you'll find yourself chronically overloaded, often to the point of desperation. Many women have an especially hard time with the "N" word. Practicing in front of a mirror can be a helpful way to overcome this problem. Role-play this exchange between two sisters for instance:

*Janis:*   So you're going to do Thanksgiving this year, right, Tracy?

---

| | |
|---|---|
| *Tracy:* | Well, I hadn't planned on it. |
| *Janis:* | Oh, you have to! You're so good at it. |
| *Tracy:* | You're good at it, too. |
| *Janis:* | Not like you. Nobody makes a turkey like you do. Mom's always saying. And your stuffing. |
| *Tracy:* | I don't think I can do it this year, Janis. I've got enough on my plate as it is. I'm in school and I've got the kids and it's just too much. |
| *Janis:* | I'll help. |
| *Tracy:* | How about if I help you? I really think it's your turn this year. |
| *Janis:* | You want to think about it? |
| *Tracy:* | No. I've made up my mind. This year it's your turn. |

Saying "no" wasn't easy for Tracy and it may not be easy for you. It may take a lot of practice, depending on how out-of-the-habit you've gotten. But don't give up. You can do it!

## Anger Management

If you haven't mastered the fine art of assertiveness, then you probably will find yourself in quite a few situations where you feel angry. Even if you have mastered the fine art of assertiveness, anger will still surface in your life and you will still have to deal with angry feelings now and then. Some people deal with anger by repressing it. Maybe they'll get a headache or become constipated or do something to their own bodies that their own bodies don't deserve. Other people will deal with anger by displacing it. They've had a run-in with their boss and instead of asserting themselves in the situation, they'll go home and have a fight with a spouse or with the kids or hurt an innocent bystander in some way. Still others may walk around with anger until it builds up into rage, and then the rage comes out in wildly explosive and highly inappropriate ways. We've all heard of road rage and airport rage, and the outcome of those reactions can often be frighteningly intense and even, in some situations, tragic.

So how do we manage our anger in ways that are effective? Here are some thoughts from your colleagues.

⌣ **Anger is a normal part of life.** You don't have to look at anger like it's some kind of monster, some dragon that's been let out of the cage. But if you don't have an okay relationship with your own anger, it might become a dragon let out of a cage. So the important thing is for you to be able to take your "anger temperature." How angry are you? On a scale of 1 to 10, are you a four? A seven? Are you off the charts at 11? If you're in the boiling point zone, you have to take some emergency actions and make sure that you're not going to do something you regret like drive your car through the other person's front door. Some actions, once they've been taken, cannot be undone and the consequences can be really life-changing, for both you and the object of your anger.

꙳ **If I'm really raging,** I'll force myself to breathe deeply. Deep breathing is the best response to that kind of anger. All that oxygen flowing into my body has a very beneficial effect on me. Make sure, though, to deep breathe. That means breathing from the diaphragm, bringing it up from the gut. Shallow breathing isn't going to help.

꙳ **Somebody, at some point** in your life, must have told you to count to 10 when you get angry. It's a cliché but you know what? It makes a lot of sense. The idea is to give yourself some breathing room, and if you count to 10, you might not say the first stupid thing that comes into your head.

꙳ **When I'm really, really mad,** I pick a word and I just repeat it, over and over again, until I come down a little. For some people, the word could be as simple as "relax." I like to say "easy" to myself: it's what I might say to a wild horse I'm trying to tame. Taming myself when I feel that way is my first priority.

꙳ **The same way** you can use guided imagery for anxiety relief you can use for anger management. Like if you've just had a huge blowout with your room-mate, for instance, who's accused you of using too much toilet paper or whatever, you can remove yourself from the apartment, go across the street to the park or the coffee shop, and play in your mind a movie of yourself at the beach, if that's a favorite place for you to be. Picture yourself lying on a blanket, on the sand, listening to your favorite song, and staring up at the skywriting in the bright blue sky . . . whatever makes you feel calmer and more rational.

🌀 **I'm a yoga person,** so if I find myself in a situation where I've gone off the deep end, anger-wise, I'll get out my mat and I'll do some movements. It always helps me. If you've got some physical activity that helps you that way, by all means make sure that you do it.

🌀 **What I've learned to do** when I think I'm veering out of control is to reframe what's happening. I used to be the kind of person who, when things were going wrong, would say stuff like, "It's horrible. It's terrible. It's the end of the world." What I learned to do was to substitute a different and more specific vocabulary for all that nonsense I was saying to myself. Now, I'll use phrases like, "It's frustrating" or "It's annoying" or "I'm disappointed" or "I'm upset." These are still ways to acknowledge that I'm feeling bad about something, but they're not end-of-the-world words.

🌀 **I try to stay away from** certain "hot-button" words like "Never" or "Always." Those are the kinds of very charged words—"You never do anything right"; "I'm always waiting for you"—that only make things worse.

🌀 **Sometimes, you can put the fire out** by just using a little logic. You can tell yourself, for instance, that the world is not out to get you. The world doesn't even know who you are. You know the bumper sticker "Think globally, act locally?" Well, we could all use a bumper sticker that says "Think locally, act locally." Put the global out of your head altogether.

ॐ **Listen.** Listen, listen, listen. If you actually can get yourself to listen to what the other person has to say, half of the arguments you have probably never would have happened in the first place.

ॐ **Humor or just plain silliness** is to anger what a pin is to a balloon. It just takes the air out of it. When I get really angry with someone, like my boss, who's such a clown, I make up these caricatures of him. I draw him like he's a potato head, which is sort of what he looks like anyway. I laugh till I feel better, but I remember not to leave the drawings around.

ॐ **I try to prevent fights** by avoiding those things that I know are going to set me off. Like my son's room. He's 15 and he's an Olympic-caliber slob. I mean really world class. I've found cupcakes under his pillow, and looking under his bed is like being sucked into this black hole. But I pick my battles. If I didn't, I'd be fighting with him 24/7. So you know what I do? I keep his door closed. It works.

# Stress Relievers

Now that we've looked at some of the "big picture" sources and issues around stress, let's focus in on some of the many ways that you can control and relieve your stress so that it won't get the best of you. Remember that in our modern world and in the field you've chosen, you're never going to be completely stress-free. To achieve that goal, you might have to become a monk living in a monastery in the mountains somewhere, although these days, there really is no immunity from stress wherever you are. But these tips from your colleagues will certainly help you balance the scale when it feels like it's going out of whack.

☾ **There's no better stress reliever** than deep breathing. It calms you and energizes you at the same time. You can do it anywhere, anytime. It doesn't cost anything. It can lower blood pressure. Now you're going to ask me how you can breathe deeply when you're feeling stressed and can't get a deep breath, right? Good question. It's something you learn how to do. Go to a yoga class and find out.

☾ **I do deep breathing** with a twist. When I'm stressed, I tell myself to "breathe in the good" as I'm breathing in and "breathe out the bad" as I'm breathing out. You'd be amazed how much of a stress-buster this can be.

☾ **My cure for stress** is sleep. I know a lot of people can't sleep when they're stressed, but for me, it's the opposite. I make a point of getting into bed before 10 P.M. and listening to some Celtic music. That way, I'm good for eight hours.

❧ **In our society,** we're bombarded by ads for drugs that are there to take the edge off stress. I'm not knocking those drugs, as long as people carefully follow doctor's orders, but getting bombed after work or cutting out of the salon every hour for a smoke are unacceptable antistress responses, as far as I'm concerned. They only cause more stress over the long run. To me, the way to deal with stress is to find a few minutes every day to go inside of myself and to connect with my spiritual side. Whether that is achieved by meditation, prayer, yoga, a walk in the woods or in the park, or simply by deep breathing is up to each person. But do it.

❧ **A lot of stress** comes as a result of people not having good problem-solving skills. I watch people walk around eating themselves up about some unsolved problem when they could just as well figure things out with a little deductive reasoning and logic.

❧ **You want to know how** I beat stress? By giving myself goodies. Whenever I've come through a rough patch where I'm running myself ragged, I reward myself with a special treat. Maybe it's a fruit smoothie, maybe it's a half hour in a bubble bath, maybe it's a nap, or maybe it's a nap with a friend!

❧ **Laughing helps.** When I'm stressed out, I turn off the news on the car radio and I put on a comedy tape. When I laugh, I can feel the stress flying out of my body. It's hilarious.

❧ **Crying helps.** I don't mean wallowing in self-pity. I mean putting on some great old movie where the heroine is going to die but doesn't tell her lover until it's over, and I've got four handkerchiefs going and I can feel all that stress just exiting my body in the form of tears.

❧ **When I know I'm going to be** in a high-stress situation, I make sure that I get my B vitamins and calcium. The stuff that people shovel into their mouths when they're stressed—colas, fried foods, chips, junk food, white sugar—just puts more stress on their bodies. Eating a lot of raw foods will help get through a stress situation.

❧ **When I'm stressed,** I steer clear of caffeine. Taking in a lot of caffeine when I'm stressed is like throwing fat on the fire. I reach for the chamomile instead.

❧ **You want to know what** will take away half the stress in your life? Ending unhealthy relationships, if that's what you're into. I know it's not that easy, but it's got to be done, and you might as well bite the bullet and do it. Unhealthy relationships are the number one leading cause of stress. They're toxic!

❧ **A good way to reduce stress** in your life is to reduce the noise level. Turn off the hip-hop. Turn off the TV. Enjoy the quiet. Listen to calming music. We live with such a loud soundtrack in our lives, it's really a problem.

**❂ The world is a stressful place.** You turn on the news and you hear all about war and people dying and the economy going belly up. If you can't handle that kind of stress, then steer clear of it. Does that mean you're an ostrich putting your head in the sand? Well, if you are and if that's what you need to do to survive, at least for a while, then so be it.

**❂ Stop smoking!**

**❂ You want to know my secret** weapon against stress? Vacations! Seriously, a lot of us forget to take them, particularly if we're working for ourselves. Some of us are lucky if we take a week a year. That's nuts. The therapeutic effect of a vacation can be enormous. Even a day off, when feeling really stressed out, can make a world of difference. Spend the day bicycling or pack a picnic and head for the beach.

**❂ For me, it's hobbies.** I weave. It transports me away from every care I have in the world. I absolutely adore it.

**❂ I look for the gift in things.** It's a kind of Buddhist mentality, but it says that no matter what happens, there is always a gift to be found in the event. If your mother dies, the gift might be that you are freed up to see the better parts of who she was. If you lose your job, the gift might be that you are forced to go out and look for another one and maybe find a better one. It's just a way of thinking that focuses on opportunity, not loss.

ℭ **You're not going to have much stress relief** in your life if you don't have a strong support system to get you through the rough times. For some people, that means family, but other people make friends who are like family and are always there for them, in the good times and the bad.

ℭ **Live within your means.** If you're spending more than you're making and running up crazy credit card bills, you're going to feel stress. Boy, are you going to feel stress. Is that extra sweater or pair of shoes really worth it?

As we've said, don't expect to completely eliminate stress from your life. The goal is to manage it and to control it so it doesn't take over. One way to keep stress under control is to make sure that you're as organized and on top of things as you need to be. In the next chapter, that's what we'll be focusing on.

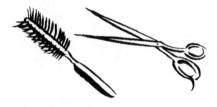

# Chapter 10

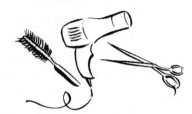

## GETTING ORGANIZED

*"Be prepared."*
*"Neatness counts."*
*"Dot your i's and cross your t's."*

**T**hese expressions, which you've probably heard from parents, teachers, and other authority figures all your life, may make you crazy. They may be exactly the opposite of how you think and how you view the world. Maybe you see yourself as a free spirit, a square peg in a world of round holes, a person who likes to do things your own way. But no matter how free-spirited you are, or how talented and artistic, the fact is that when you are working in a field like cosmetology, you need to have a certain level of organizational skills to get you through your day. And as a student, you need those skills more than ever.

Think back to grade school when you were always forgetting your pencils, your books, and your lunch. Your teacher got pretty annoyed with you, didn't she?

Chances are, there was a little boy or girl in your class who never forgot anything, who always had the books, the pencils, the lunch. That student got an A, right? And now the time has come in your life when you want to be the one getting the recognition for being the best. That requires that you stop forgetting things and start remembering what's important.

Being highly organized won't make you the best but it certainly will help. Being disorganized means that you're wasting too much time and will probably have to repeat your tasks. Do you really have the time for that at this point in your life?

Getting organized and managing your time is part art, part science, and part pure determination. Even if it is not in your basic nature to be terribly organized, you can still make significant improvements in that department. In this chapter, you will be reading a lot of tips on the subject of organization. We hope that you'll start thinking about how you can put these ideas into practice.

## Time Management

There's no time like the present to start talking about time and what it means to you. Time is a very sensitive issue. People who are chronically late wear out the patience of others, and there are few professions more time-sensitive than cosmetology where you are being asked to stick to a schedule that impacts on clients and coworkers. Cosmetologists who cannot manage their time run the risk of becoming cosmetologists with all the time in the world; in other words, out-of-work cosmetologists.

Even before you become a licensed cosmetologist, your life as a student will demand that you think about how best to use your time. There are only so many hours in the day, and chances are you're juggling school, work obligations, and family. If you fail to make the most of your time, you run the risk of falling seriously behind, and the more you fall behind, the harder it gets to catch up.

↻ **Time was always a big issue** in my family growing up. Every Sunday we went to church, and every Sunday my mom was always late getting us there. She and my dad would wind up fighting, which I don't think was the point of going to church exactly. Growing up that way, I had a hard time finding my balance. Sometimes I'd be very late; sometimes I'd be very early to try to make up for those times I was late. I finally wound up going to a counselor who taught me about my "inner organizer." It's like a natural clock you carry around inside. Some people have a nice quiet clock that keeps good time; others have clocks that tick loud and fast and that don't always work. When I found out what my clock was like, I could learn to listen to it and let it guide me.

↻ **In high school, I was famous** for coming to class late. My English teacher used to call me "Jenny Come Lately" because my name's Jenny and apparently there's some old expression about "Johnny Come

Lately." But I didn't come late because I didn't care, the way some kids do. I came late because I had a hard time organizing myself and getting myself together to move from one class to another. I still do. I'm still leaving stuff in one class and having to run back to get it so that I'm late for the next class. It used to be kind of cute or funny or something when I was younger. Now that I'm 31, it's just a pain for my teachers, for the other students in my classes, and most of all for me.

๑ **When you're a student,** it's important to put some kind of time management system into place. I mean, there's a lot to keep track of and I don't want to be one of those people who is always trying to catch up. On the other hand, I don't want to be one of those people who walks around with a clipboard and a stopwatch like maybe I'm some kind of efficiency expert and I can get all the trains to run on time. That's not me either. The point is to create a system that reflects the way I like to live. Some people get off on living by the clock; others need a more flexible system with blocks of "free time" set aside. That's not to say that these people can't be organized and efficient. It's just a question of style.

๑ **As far as I'm concerned,** time management begins with *prioritization*. Between my three teenagers and going back to school, I have to figure out what I can do effectively, what I can try to do, and what I have to admit to myself that I simply can't do. If I can get the entire first group done and a good chunk of the second, then I sort of feel that the third will take care of itself.

Ↄ **If you're trying to find a way** to manage your time, it helps to stop thinking of time as the enemy. People are always worrying about time: how it's slipping away, how there's never enough of it. Sometimes people worry about time so much that they can't even see the gifts of time that they get unexpectedly. Whereas one person might see a cancelled appointment as something to get all upset over, others might see it as this present that has dropped in their lap. Maybe that hour will be an opportunity to finally clean or arrange or in some other way catch up with what's been put off. Maybe that snowstorm will be a ticket to a wonderful day at home playing with the kids.

Ↄ **If you think about it,** the issue of time management is very much linked to the issue of assertiveness. If you can't say "no," then people are going to take advantage of you and your time is going to be eaten up.

Ↄ **If I really want to get things done,** I have to be direct with people almost to the point of rudeness. Someone might call me on my cell and say "Do you have a minute?" and I'm like, "No." If I don't say "no," I know I'm going to get myself into big trouble.

Ↄ **Making phone calls,** even routine ones, eats up a lot of time, so I try to return calls when people are less likely to want to shmooze. Right before lunch or at the end of the day is a good time to have short, sweet conversations with people.

Ↄ **Some people can handle interruptions** better than other people. I'm not good at it. I know that about myself, so whenever I travel anywhere, I bring the Do Not Disturb sign home with me. I've got a whole bunch of them and I use them. When I go into my room to study, I hang one from my doorknob and my kids know that it's like the law that they can't come in.

☾ **I "give" people time.** If my mother or my sister calls me at work, I say, "Okay. You've got three minutes." They may not be too crazy about that approach, but to me it's like a little gift: three minutes out of my crazy day.

# Making Lists

You may not think of yourself as a "list" sort of person, but the fact is that few of us can survive without them. Nothing compares to a "to-do" list when it comes to keeping your days under control. Whether you use a pocket calendar, an electronic organizer, a stick-it pad, or a ballpoint pen on the palm of your hand, don't leave home without it! You'll want to keep a daily to-do list for sure, but you may also find that a weekly or even monthly to-do list has a lot of benefits as well.

☾ **I find it really helpful** to review my to-do list at the same time every day. I used to do it first thing in the morning, over coffee, which was okay, but lately I've been doing it before I go to bed at night and I like that even better. I know no one is going to disturb me and so I have 10 or 15 minutes to look over my list and think in a peaceful and calm way about the day that's ahead of me.

☺ **I have one rule** I never break: I keep my to-do list to one page. If it's more than one page, that means there's too much to do on my to-do list!

☺ **A to-do list** doesn't make sense unless you prioritize it. Put the most important thing at the top of your list. In other words, Exam or Interview or Mammogram goes at the top while Cleaning the Grout Around the Bathtub goes at the bottom or gets bumped off the list altogether.

☺ **Everybody has their own way** of keeping a to-do list. Mine has two columns. One column says Hard, the other says Easy. If I know I have some easy stretches ahead of me, I can deal with the hard parts.

☺ **When you're organizing your to-do list,** keep in mind what kind of energy you have at different points of the day. Don't put the stuff that takes a lot of energy into the 4 P.M. slot, let's say, when you're dragging yourself around. If you're a real get-up-and-go personality, maybe you'll want to schedule heavy before lunch and go lighter in the afternoon. Your call.

☺ **Unless you're the kind of person** who does crossword puzzles in pen, always write your to-do list in pencil because it's going to change. Things get canceled and shuffled around all the time. Think of the to-do list as a work in progress.

꙼ **Call it a to-do list if you want,** but I like to think of it as a list of goals. I don't just write everything down that comes into my head. I write down those things that I think I stand a chance of accomplishing. I never have more than 10 items on a list in one day. If I can manage to get 10 solid things done, I consider that a very good day indeed. Nine is good too. Eight is good. Seven is fine. Five or six, I don't kick myself, but three or four means I'm sleepwalking and probably need to recharge with some protein, a massage, or a day off. Less than three or four means I'm getting the flu or getting married or something like that.

꙼ **When I make up a to-do list,** I try to bunch certain things together in a way that makes sense. Like geographically, for instance. It's the same principle as when I make a shopping list. I put all the dairy together and all the fruits and vegetables together and so on, so that I'm not running down one aisle for the cottage cheese and another aisle for the baked beans and another aisle for an avocado and then back to the dairy section for the eggs.

꙼ **Here's a tip that's so obvious** it's almost embarrassing, but I'll say it anyway. Finish one task before going on to the next. In other words, if you've prioritized your to-do list, as you should have, don't go on to the number four priority until you've got the number one priority sorted away.

꙼ **Making a list without prioritizing** doesn't make a whole lot of sense. So how do you figure out priorities? Here's what I do. I ask myself what good or bad thing is going to happen if I do or do not get something done. If I don't get an assignment done on time, I may get a lower grade. Bad thing. If I do get an assignment done on time, I stand a better chance of getting a good grade and I'll have plenty of time to get tomorrow's assignment done in time. Good thing.

ℒ **Look, we're all human,** and we all run behind now and then. If you do, don't make yourself crazy (and please don't make those around you crazy!). Just carry over the item you didn't get to onto tomorrow's list. But make sure you don't just add onto tomorrow's list so that now you've got 13 on your list instead of a manageable nine or ten.

ℒ **Check off your to-do list** as you go along. It feels good to check those little buggers off and to see how much you got done!

ℒ **Before I went back to school,** I just kept a daily to-do list. I was working in a child care center and frankly, I didn't have as much to keep on top of as I do now. As a cosmetology student, I've got a ton of things to keep track of so I've started keeping a weekly to-do list in addition to my daily to-do list. This way, I can bite off bigger chunks of time and try to bring some perspective to them. If I have a project due a month ahead, I can see it coming on the horizon. Next step is the monthly list!

ℒ **The same way that I prioritize** my daily to-do list is how I prioritize my weekly list. For example, I tell myself that I can only watch three hours of TV a week no matter what. I just don't have time for more and it turns my brain to jelly. So I pick my programs carefully.

⟳ **Everybody's got their own method,** but my "sanity secret" is to schedule in at least one block of free time a day. No matter how packed the day is that's coming up, I factor in free time. That way, I've got protection in case something unexpected comes along like car trouble, baby-sitting trouble, or whatever. And something unexpected always does come up!

⟳ **Not only are to-do lists valuable,** but also now that I use a real organizer, I see how many other great aids there are at my disposal. My organizer, for instance, has an insert that helps me keep track of expenses, and my girlfriend uses one of those electronic organizers that practically runs her life.

⟳ **I always carry a pen and pad** with me wherever I go. I never know when a good idea might strike. I never depend on my ability to "remember it later."

# The Lost and Found of Time

If you keep close tabs on how you use your time over the course of a few weeks, chances are you'll be shocked by how much of it slips through your fingers. All of us can save hours a week just by becoming aware of certain little shortcuts and "fast ones" we can pull on old Father Time.

There's no end to the ways you can save time when you start paying attention to your use of it. The following tips will give you some ideas of ways to own your time again in all the many areas of your life.

## Shopping and Cooking

✪ **Cooking can eat up** much too much time, but you don't have to let it. You can still be considered a really good cook just using a repertoire of meals that you can cook in 30 minutes or less. You'll find all kinds of cookbooks out there that specialize in good, fast cooking.

✪ **Double quantities when cooking** whenever you can. If you freeze away the extras, you'll have two or three meals for the "time price" of one.

✪ **I keep a shopping list** with a pencil on a string on the refrigerator door. Whenever I use something up, I write it on the list. Then I go to the store with a friend or one of my kids, tear the list in half, and we meet back at the checkout having done the job in half the time.

✪ **My trick when it comes to shopping** is to always shop in the same supermarket. Supermarkets today are so huge that if you go to a new one you're unfamiliar with, it will take you three times as long.

When I go to the same one all the time, I know exactly where the onions, light bulbs, toilet paper, and cat food are, like I know the back of my hand.

↻ **If I'm shopping and I see something** I love, like a blouse that's really right for me or whatever and that's not going to go out of style, I'll buy two, if I can afford it. I know that when one wears out, I'll still have the other and I won't have to spend the time to go out shopping for the perfect blouse.

↻ **I do a lot of shopping** on the Internet. I get great prices and I don't have to drive to a mall and look for a parking place. A lot of the stores you go to in the mall have Internet sites with special Internet bargains, too.

## Around the House

↻ **I'm the president** of the international "I Hate Cleaning" society. The same way I prioritize my to-do list is how I prioritize my housecleaning. I figure out what needs to be done on a daily basis (picking up dirty clothes from the floor), on a weekly basis (cleaning the bathrooms, throwing out garbage, a little light vacuuming), what needs to be done monthly (I don't know, changing the linen?), and yearly (turning the mattress? washing the windows? Yeah, right!).

↻ **I keep cheap** handheld vacuum cleaners on every level of the house. I hardly ever take out the big vacuum except maybe if company is coming.

In our house, everyone has a cubby. That's where coats, hats, gloves, and shoes go. As for me, I always keep my keys and wallet in the same place. I used to be less careful about that and I'd spend hours every week looking for things and dealing with extra stress that I needed like a hole in the head.

One of the things that used to eat up a lot of my time was looking for stuff. Scissors, scotch tape, screwdriver; everyday stuff like that. Then I had this brainstorm. I could buy four screwdrivers at $.99 apiece and I could keep them in strategic parts of the house. Same for scissors, tape, and all those other little things I'm always misplacing. It's great!

## Laundry

If you have kids, the rule is white socks only! I don't want to hear any whining about how they have to have polka dots or little teddy bears on their socks. Everyone wears white and all things are equal.

Consider a sleeping bag for your kids' beds instead of linen. They'll be just as happy, laundering will be easier, and there are no beds to make up.

## Home Maintenance

Silhouette your tools on a pegboard so you'll know just where everything goes.

If you're always in a panic looking for warranties and appliance manuals and stuff like that, do what I did. Get a three-ring binder, punch holes in those important papers, and keep them all together where you will always know where to find them.

☙ **It's a little thing,** but it makes me crazy: the amount of time it takes to untangle stuff like electric cords, Christmas tree lights, garden hoses, and whatever else has the capacity to get tangled. Now I put everything like that on reels and it saves me a lot of grief.

## Travel

☙ **As a working cosmetologist,** I do a lot of shows, which means I travel all the time. So I keep a master list of everything I need to take with me: my makeup, shampoo, alarm clock, pharmaceuticals. Before I leave the house on any trip, I check each item off on my master list and I almost never get caught without the things I need.

☙ **I like to keep** an extra cosmetic bag packed just for travel so it's always ready to go.

☙ **If I can,** I get foreign currency ahead of time.

☙ **Consider using a travel agent** to make travel plans. Chances are, it won't cost you any more and you'll save tons of time not waiting on the telephone to talk to some person at an airline.

## Miscellaneous Time Savers

☙ **I try to cut down** on all unnecessary trips. For instance, if I'm out shopping and my gas tank is still half full, I'll fill it anyway so I won't have to make a special trip at some other point just to get gas.

☾ **Have you discovered** automated banking? It rocks!

☾ **I relaxed my standards.** In the past, if I wanted to have friends over, I'd feel that I'd have to make a beautiful dinner. Well, you can imagine how many friends I had to dinner, given my schedule and that mind-set. Now when I have friends over, everyone brings a dish. It's fun and it's easy.

☾ **Make the best use of your commute.** If you're in walking distance to work, walk the walk and make this into your exercise time. If you're sitting on a bus or a subway, you might take this time to learn a new skill—knitting? the rules of bridge?—or you might further organize your to-do list or catch up on some much-needed sleep. If you're driving, check out books-on-tape. You can learn so much about so many different things while you're stuck in traffic.

☾ **Once you're out working** in the field, if the idea of hiring help makes sense with your budget, give this option careful consideration. Many of us are relentless "do-it-yourselfers" and feel that it is too much of a luxury or a cop-out to hire someone to clean our house, fix our leaky faucets, or change a pane of broken glass. It is all well and good to do these things yourself, but there are only so many hours in the day, and if you can charge $50 for an hour of your time servicing a client, it may make sense to hire a housecleaner who charges $25 an hour for her work.

🔗 **Buy a phone answering machine** if you don't already have one. That way, you can monitor incoming calls and decide when and if you want to take them. For instance, if you come home and you need an hour to be by yourself or with your family, you can get back to Aunt Dottie at some other point. She'll understand and what she doesn't know won't hurt her. Another option is to consider getting rid of your answering machine. That way, you'll never have to return a call!

🔗 **I like to take advantage** of down time. For me, it begins first thing in the morning. I set my alarm a half hour before I actually have to get up and then I luxuriate in bed before I have to confront another hectic day ahead of me.

🔗 **If you have kids,** carpool, carpool, carpool! It's insane to live any other way.

---

### Beating the Morning Madness

Mornings are the hardest for many people, particularly if you live in a house with many people (or any people other than you!). Here are some ways that your peers have found to make the mornings go smoother:

✂ Teach your family to pack school bags, briefcases, the baby's diaper bag, and whatever else is needed for the day the night before and put them by the door.

---

✂ Lay out your work clothing the night before. If you're really good, you might want to use Sunday night to arrange your work wardrobe for the week. It takes a load off to know that you have five days of clean, ironed clothing ahead of you.

✂ Keep a chalkboard, a dry-erase board, or a pencil and pad by the door for any last minute messages or notes.

✂ A bowl of coins goes a long way toward commutes, tolls, school lunches, money for a newspaper, and so forth. Make a routine of emptying your pockets into the bowl at night. It beats picking up pennies from the floor when you take your pants off.

✂ Either you or your admirably self-sufficient children can pack school lunches the night before and stick them in the fridge.

Okay, now that you're communicating effectively, handling stress, feeling organized, and whatever else you've learned from this book so far, let's move on to a subject that has enormous impact on all of our lives: money.

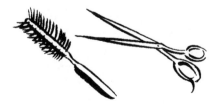

# Chapter 11

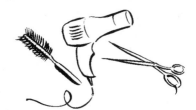

## ALL ABOUT MONEY

*"Money frees you from doing things you dislike. Since I dislike doing nearly everything, money comes in handy."*
—*Groucho Marx*

*"Money is better than poverty, if only for financial reasons."*
—*Woody Allen*

*"My problem lies in reconciling my gross habits with my net income."*

—*Erroll Flynn*

Y ou've just read what three Hollywood legends had to say about money. Food for thought, to be sure, but, of course, there is a great deal more to be said on this matter that rules people's lives as much as they let it. So let's begin.

One of the reasons you may have enrolled in cosmetology school is because you had reason to believe that this is a field that will pay well. Certainly, there is considerable money to be made in cosmetology, but that money is still way off in your future, isn't it? At the moment, you've got bills, bills, and more bills.

As strapped as you sometimes feel in the here and now, however, you should realize that money is going to be something you'll have to deal with throughout your life, whether you're rich, poor, or in between. As a student of cosmetology, you've been hearing a lot about the importance of continuing education. There are always new fashions and technological advances, and you have to stay on top of things. The same is true of money. You have to regard money as an important subject for lifelong learning. So while this overview may serve as a nice way to open up the discussion, its purpose is really to inspire you to do more reading and research on your own.

# The Psychology of Money

Money is a subject that never seems to be neutral. It carries a positive or negative charge, or sometimes both at the same time. As we grow up, our families give us all kinds of different messages about money.

"Money makes the world go around."

"Money is the root of all evil."

"Marry a rich man."

"Get a regular paycheck."

"Never tell anybody what you make."

Our task, as we mature into adulthood, is to process these messages and come up with something that we can feel comfortable living with. Let's see how your fellow cosmetology students are processing.

☾ **Some of us** come from families with diverse religious cultures and beliefs. In my family, money was our religion. My parents owned a furniture store and they were there, both of them, 12 hours a day. The only thing they ever talked about or cared about was money. The only presents they ever gave were money. The idea of giving a doll or a pretty hair ribbon would have made no sense to them whatsoever. They gave money, and whoever got it could do what they wanted with it.

☾ **I come from a family** where the worst thing in the world you could do was talk about money. It was better you should talk about sex. To me, it made money into this incredible unknowable thing, and it's taken me half of my adult life to realize that money is just a tool. If you know how to use it, you can get things done. It's not a mystery. It's a reality.

☾ **My family was very old-fashioned.** The men made the money; the women did everything else. When I got married, I kept up the tradition. My husband was an ophthalmologist and made lots of money. My job was to make a beautiful home, and let me tell you, you could have eaten off my floor. Then, on our 20th anniversary, my husband divorced me. Suddenly, I had a whole lot of learning to do about money. I was always good with hair so it seemed like a good direction. And it has been. This skill has allowed me to rebuild my life in not very much time at all, thank goodness.

✑ **Living in the United States** in the 21st century means living in a consumer culture. Sure, there are some people who live an alternate lifestyle and don't buy into all that, but for the most part, we're being bombarded by advertising and credit card offers. I grew up in the Ukraine and it was a whole different story there. When I came to the United States, I felt like I was coming to some gigantic fair where everything was buy, buy, buy. Now that I've been here 15 years, I can step back a little. Now I try to be careful not to care too much about material things at the expense of things that are nonmaterial like nature and love and spirituality.

✑ **We live in the richest society** in history. And we also live in a society where the gap between the rich and the poor is greater than it's ever been. Being rich today doesn't mean having millions. It means having billions. In this kind of environment, you run the risk of equating material worth with inner worth. The more money a person has, the "better" or more "successful" you figure that person has to be. But being well off and being a good human being are not one and the same. The most successful human being I ever knew was my father, a baker. Why? Because he loved people and people loved him, and everything he made with his own two hands was indescribably delicious.

🌊 **When it comes to money,** you have to strike a balance you're comfortable with. How much of your life are you willing to dedicate to making money? How much time away from your personal life are you prepared to give up? I remember once reading about this guy who resigned as the CEO of a large company so he'd have more time for his private life. He said, "I never heard of anybody saying at the end of their life that they regretted the time they spent with their family."

🌊 **I have a brother** who's a financial whiz—he made a ton of money on the stock market—and he tells me that money is a game. I mean, he's not saying that it's all play money, but his point is that you should have some fun with money. He says that no matter what you earn, you should use part of it, even a tiny part, to grow in some exciting way.

## The Financial Pyramid

No doubt you've heard of the Food Pyramid. You probably studied it at some point in health class. Well, there's such a thing as a Financial Pyramid, too, which offers a graphic representation of your lifetime financial goals. At the base are your Values and Goals: do you want to retire at 45? Become a philanthropist? Live in a camper? Figure it out, and when you do, construct your base. The next step represents your basic living expenses: food, shelter, clothing, transportation, and the like. Before you spend money on other things, you have to meet those needs. Once you've budgeted for basics, you can climb up to the next layer of Savings, Credit, and Insurance. From there, you might move on to Owning a Home. At the very top is Investing for the Future, which has to do with your children's college tuitions, your retirement, and so forth. The Financial Pyramid helps you prioritize your goals and allot your resources where they are needed most.

## Budgeting

Some people have an allergic reaction to the word "budgeting." They think of it as an activity for other people but not for themselves. The reality, however, is that we all need to budget. Even people who make huge sums of money need to keep budgetary concerns in mind. There are plenty of tragic tales out there about rock stars and movie stars who made wheelbarrows full of money but lived so extravagantly that nothing was left when the lights dimmed. Money can be a real stimulant, like alcohol or cocaine, and when it's new to you, you have to learn how to integrate it into your life and not become a "user." Budgeting is the tool that helps you keep your spending under control. Let's have a look at what your colleagues have to say on the subject of budgeting.

☯ **Most people think of budgeting** as a matter of dollars and cents: what comes in and what goes out. But budgeting is more than that. The real value of budgeting is that it helps you focus on your goals. You see exactly what you need to do to reach your goal and how long it will take you. For instance, if you have $100 a month left over after all your monthly expenses, you might want to save $80 of that money each month and put $20 of it toward the sound system you want to buy. In a certain amount of time, you will have saved enough money to buy that system, which is different than just putting the purchase on a credit card and paying it off at 23 percent.

☯ **If you're going to get started** with budgeting— and everyone should—you should have some understanding of what income and expenses are. Some people think of income only as your salary, but it's more than that. It could be an allowance from your parents or spouse or alimony or child support payments or welfare payments or food stamps. It could include student financial aid and tax refunds. Gifts are income. If your Uncle Morris gives you $100 at Christmas, that's income. Interest earned on savings is income, too, as are dividends earned on investments.

☯ **There are a few key term**s you really need to know if you're going to start getting serious about money. Like the difference between gross and net. The total amount of your income, collected from all sources, is your gross income. If you're working, your employer withholds certain amounts from your paycheck in order to pay federal and local taxes, social security (FICA), group insurance premiums, union dues, pension contributions, and other deductions. The amount of money left over is called your net income, which is, of course, less than your gross income.

꙰ **When you're budgeting,** you have to know the difference between fixed and variable expenses. Fixed expenses don't change. Your rent or mortgage payments, your utilities, telephone, car payments, and insurance payments are all fixed expenses. Variable expenses are those that come up only now and then, and are often unpredictable. If you bite down on an olive pit and break a tooth, you've got a variable expense. If your transmission goes, that's another variable expense.

꙰ **My Uncle Bernie,** my father's uncle, was an accountant, and he used to tell us—when he'd lecture us about money, which he did at every family gathering—that there was such a thing as the "Four A's of Budgeting." You *account* for your income and expenses. You *analyze* the situation after you've had a look at the numbers. You *allocate* your income, using it as you see fit. And you *adjust* your budget as necessary.

꙰ **The way to start budgeting** is to keep track of everything you spend money on at least for a couple of months. Carry around a little notepad and jot down all your expenses: buses, subways, lunch, magazines, an ice cream cone, coffee. Whenever you spend money, write it down, with the date, and don't forget to enter the purchases you make by credit card or over the Internet. They didn't come free, you know. The idea is to step back after a couple of months so that you can study your patterns. You'll get a sense of where the money went, and you may decide to make changes.

♋ **When you get a good look** at where your money's gone and you tally up the numbers, you can start to ask the hard questions. Were your expenses more than your income? Were you able to cover all your fixed expenses? Did any sudden expenses come up? Were you able to handle them? Did you pay off your credit card balance? If not, did you at least make the minimum payment? These are hard questions and a lot of people don't like to ask them, but the longer you put it off, the bigger the hole you're digging for yourself.

♋ **It's easy to panic** when you first start budgeting. Even when you've been doing it for a while and you've gotten used to it, it can still get scary. The first thing to do—after you've take that deep breath—is to look at your fixed expenses and make sure you've got the money for them. Rent, utilities, phone, insurance: there's no room to negotiate around those expenses. If you come up short, then you can look at your variable expenses and start chopping away. Cigarettes? Now there's a no-brainer. They cost a fortune plus they give you lung cancer. Instead of that double mocha latté for $3.50, how about a good old-fashioned cup of coffee for $1? If possible, walk instead of using public transportation: the health benefits are as good as the money-saving benefits. And stay away from restaurants. This is a good time for you to enjoy some nice home cooking. Your own!

〰 **I always make sure** to factor emergency money into my budget. Like if my car breaks down and suddenly I need $300 for a new ball joint, I'd rather have some emergency money put aside than have to go to my parents or whatever. I'm sure they'd give it to me, but that would mean they'd have to do without something that month.

〰 **My dad's always after us** to save. He says that it's really a good growth thing to set your mind on something—a vacation, a couch, a car, whatever— and save for it over the long term. He says you build up a kind of discipline about your finances that's important to learn.

〰 **You have to review your budget** regularly and make changes as necessary. A raise means a change in your budget. A layoff means a change in your budget. A baby means a change in your budget. When times are good, you'll want to treat yourself to some good-ies. It's only natural. When times are not so good, you have to tighten your belt.

# Savings and Credit

Young Americans today are saving less than the generations that came before them and are running up higher credit card debts. This dangerous situation needs to be looked at and remedied. Credit card debt can quickly become very severe.

♋ **There was an old lady** who lived down the block from us. We all called her Mama Angela. She was pretty crazy but everybody loved her. She kept all her money in the piano. Everybody knew it was there, but nobody robbed her because, like I said, we all loved her. But that's living dangerously. Banks are a better idea. You've got to know things, though, when you pick a bank. Like up to what amount are the deposits insured and who insures them (Federal insurance, like FDIC, is a better risk than state insurance funds). What are the interest rates? How easy is it to get to your money? What types of accounts are offered? Don't be afraid to ask. It's your money!

♋ **Before I went to cosmetology school,** I worked as a teller, so I know all about savings accounts. There are four basic kinds: a passbook account, which you can open with very little money but it doesn't pay much in the way of interest; a money market account with interest rates that fluctuate with the market rate, but these require a minimum balance and they often restrict withdrawals; a certificate of deposit (CD) which offers the highest rates but they tie up your money for a much longer period of time; and an individual retirement account (IRA) that is used to put aside money for retirement and which carries strict penalties if you withdraw funds before you're supposed to.

☾ **You'll discover** that the more income you earn, the more types of savings account you'll need. If you're unsure about which direction to go in, check with a friend or family member you trust, or set up a meeting with a customer service representative at a bank. That's what they're there for.

☾ **I know people** who never ever use credit cards and I know people who use credit cards every time they turn around. As far as I'm concerned, there's a middle ground. Your job is to see if you can find it.

☾ **Some people just don't understand** credit. They think it's there as some kind of public service so that you can buy those leather pants you're dying to have without having to bother to wait until you save up the money for them. What some people don't realize is that anything you buy on credit will cost you more than if you paid cash for that item. Probably a lot more. You have to factor in your interest charges and they can be steep.

☾ **Some people make credit** sound like the devil's work: you've got to stay away from it. That's a little extreme. Credit can be very useful, after all. For instance, let's say you live in a wintry climate. You're going to need snow tires to get you through the winter, right? But snow tires will set you back $300 and you just don't have that kind of money right now. But you think you'll be able to pay for it over the course of the next four or five months, so you go for it. Sure, it'll cost you more in carrying charges, but it's better than sliding off the road into a tree, isn't it? The same principle doesn't apply to cashmere sweaters, however. Snow tires can be a matter of life and death. Cashmere never is.

☾ **Playing the catch-up game** around credit is exhausting and you really wind up the loser. If you accumulate a large balance and all you ever do is make the minimum monthly payment, then all you're doing is paying off interest without ever reducing the sum you've borrowed.

☾ **Be very careful** about your credit rating. If you don't pay your bills, particularly your credit card bills, your credit rating will take a nosedive and you may be unable to get a mortgage or a business loan when you need to.

☾ **All credit cards are not created equal.** When you've made the decision that you want a credit card, you need to shop around to make sure you get one that has the best features. Most important is the APR, the annual percentage rate, which is the interest you will be charged per year on the amount you finance. Some cards have astronomical APRs, up to 23 percent. You also have to pay attention to the microscopic print, which details the finance charges. These explain the interest, fees, service charges, insurance, and other variables that differ from one company to the next.

☙ **Some people don't realize** that there's a difference between a credit card—like MasterCard, Discover, or Visa—which you can pay off over time, and a charge card—like American Express and Diner's Club—which you have to pay off in full each month.

☙ **Getting credit in the first place** can be a challenge. I remember when I first applied for a loan, I was refused because I had no credit record. So how do you develop a credit record, I wondered, if no one wants to give you credit? It's a Catch-22, right? My boyfriend suggested that I take out a small installment loan—at that time we needed a new fridge—and he would cosign the loan because he had a good credit history. As I paid off the loan for a fridge, I developed a credit history, too. Plus we got married and still are, so it all worked out for the best!

☙ **Signing up for utilities** in your own name, even though the deposit can be hefty, is another good way to start up a credit history.

☙ **You should know,** if anyone ever questions your credit rating, that you have a right to see your credit record. Credit records are maintained by credit bureaus, and they can and do make mistakes. When I went to refinance my mortgage, I almost didn't get it because a credit bureau reported that I had defaulted on mortgage payments. Of course, it turned out to be a different person with the same name as me, but if I hadn't checked, it would still be following me around. For a small fee, you can see your credit record and can know who else has seen it in the past six months. If any of the information on it is incorrect, you can have it checked out and changed, with corrected copies sent to anyone who has seen the incorrect report.

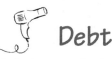

# Debt

Debt is a tough situation to be in, but keep in mind that you're not alone. Millions of Americans live with debt from year to year. In fact, it's a way of life for a lot of people.

✥ **A lot of debt** goes unnamed. For instance, there are some people who carry huge credit card debts but they act like that's not really debt. They're fooling themselves, and while they're doing it, they're getting in deeper and deeper.

✥ **Debt comes with certain telltale signs** you should pay attention to. Do you pay only the minimum on your credit cards each month? Do you juggle bills, skipping some to pay others? Are you gripped by panic every time an unexpected major expense comes up like a major car repair? Do you moonlight or depend on overtime to make ends meet? Do you borrow from family or friends? If any of the above sounds familiar, you'll want to make changes so that you can regain some control over the situation.

🌀 **I was in huge debt** for a long time and this is what I did. I called up the credit card companies and all my other creditors and I worked out a schedule for paying off the debt. Your creditors are usually pretty responsive to something like that, because they're worried about not seeing any of the money and they usually listen to whatever you offer. Another thing you can do is consolidation: putting all your debt under one roof and working out a real plan to take care of it. If you ask around, you'll be sure to find out about reputable credit consolidation companies that can help you organize your debt payoff.

🌀 **If you're seriously in debt,** get serious about resolving the problem. Contact an organization whose express purpose is to help people get out of debt. American Consumer Credit Counseling and the National Foundation for Consumer Credit are two organizations that provide credit-counseling services, either free or for a very small fee.

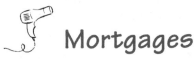

# Mortgages

Mortgages are a form of debt, buy they can work in your behalf in the sense that they can offer significant tax benefits.

☙ **If you're buying a house,** check out interest-only mortgages. These are completely tax-deductible for the first 10 years of the mortgage. In other words, you'll be able to write off your complete monthly payment. Plus, if you prepay the principle at any point, you'll not only lower your monthly payment but you'll shorten the mortgage period. This is in contrast to a fixed mortgage where the payment remains the same and you just shorten the period.

☙ **The thing you've got to be careful about** with the interest-only mortgages is that it's only interest-free for the first 10 years. After that, it turns into a 15-year amortized mortgage.

☙ **Keep in mind** that a low monthly mortgage payment can free up money for investments in the stock market or wherever. Or you might decide to put some of the extra money into home improvements, increasing the value of your property and, in turn, increasing your equity.

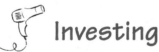

# Investing

Down the road a bit, you may find yourself with some extra money. Depending on the economic climate, one thing you might decide to do is invest it in the stock market.

☙ **One thing we've all learned** from the dot-com experience is that you've got to be really careful when you approach the market. You should only buy a stock after careful research: your research. You want to look closely at the stock's 12-month price history and its profits and earnings ratio before buying.

ॐ **Every stock** has a high and a low. When you buy a stock, you need to know whether you're buying at high or selling at low.

ॐ **My financial advisor** told me that as an investor, I shouldn't be buying and selling all the time. That's what traders do. As an investor, I should set up a long-term portfolio that takes into account my goals and my risk tolerance, and I shouldn't let the little day-to-day changes affect my long-term time frame.

ॐ **One lesson I was taught** by my cousin who's a stockbroker is that most people sell the stocks that are going up without thinking about their continued growth over the long run, and hold onto the ones that aren't going down, thinking they'll do better. He told me it should be the other way around.

ॐ **I've done well** in the market and one reason is because I was well taught. My boyfriend, who's in the financial community, taught me how important it is to study the fundamentals of a company before you buy into it. You have to look at the management, at whether the company dominates the market, if they're in the number one, number two, or number three position, and what kind of investment they make in research and development (R&D), which is how they're preparing for the future. If you do this research and things come up looking good, it's unlikely you'll go too far wrong. At least, I haven't so far. Knock wood.

☙ **The best thing I ever did** for my financial picture was to join an investment club. There are eight of us and we've pooled our money to hire an advisor who consults with us occasionally. We're doing great!

☙ **The key to investing,** as far as I'm concerned, is diversification. Never ever put all your eggs in one basket.

☙ **It's up to each individual investor** to determine the level of risk that he is comfortable with. Your stockbroker can't determine that for you. You have to figure it out for yourself and then strike a comfortable balance in your portfolio.

☙ **Personally, I look into more defensive types** of securities and I encourage others to do the same. I buy utilities, food groups, and basic companies that are always going to be there, in good times and bad. That's just my philosophy.

☙ **We've had the era** of sexy stocks. Remember all the dot.coms? Now I'm looking at tax-free municipal bonds. Okay, highway construction may not be all that sexy, but investing in these municipal bonds is a relatively safe bet. At the very least, they can help diversify an otherwise risky portfolio and I'll save money at tax time since the interest is free from federal, state, and local taxes.

This tour through the subject of money has been the barest of beginnings. Again, it's up to you to keep learning. The more you learn, the better you should be able to do with your investments and with finances in general.

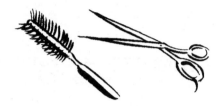

# Chapter 12

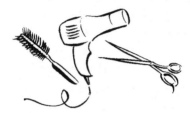

## MOVING AHEAD

Here you are, up to your necks in school responsibilities. You've got material to master, exams to pass, and plenty on your plate. It's never too early, however, to start thinking about that time, not too far ahead, when you're going to be out there, pounding the pavement, looking for a great job. You've probably been there before, knocking on doors and hoping that someone will hire you. But this time is different. This time you've got something very solid on your résumé—cosmetology school—and you're ready to run with it.

But instead of running, maybe you ought to slow down a bit and read about the best ways to undertake your job search. The tips in this chapter have been collected from cosmetology students like yourself who have all gone on to jobs. They haven't all found their dream job right off, but they're all working, learning, making money, and building a name for themselves in their chosen profession. The good news—the *very* good news—is that no matter how gloomy the economy is, there always seems to be a demand for new cosmetologists. In fact, the trend over the last few decades is that there are more jobs available than there are trained people to fill them. What could be better?

## Preparing for Licensure

Your first step in seeking employment is to make sure that you have the right credentials, and no credential is more important that the one you'll receive from having passed your state licensing examination. This examination is the stuff of many student nightmares, but it needn't be. If you have applied yourself in cosmetology school, you will be prepared. Follow the tips below and you should perform well on the actual examination.

↷ **It's a big day,** that exam. Imagine going for the gold at the Olympics or taking the stage for your Broadway debut. What would you do? Get yourself into shape, of course. You would train. You would eat well. You would exercise regularly during the weeks before the test and get plenty of sleep. You would build on a solid foundation of taking care of yourself.

↷ **On the day of the exam,** or even the night before, try to relax. Don't cram. By then, it'll be too late to make much difference anyway, and you'll only wind up making yourself more nervous than you have to be. A little nervousness is to be expected, but don't do a whole number on yourself.

✆ **A few practical tips:** find out where the exam is and visit the location the day before you're due. You don't want to get lost and have all that stress to deal with on the actual day of the exam.

✆ **Dress comfortably** on exam day, in layers, so you can add on or throw off as the temperature demands. Wear a watch so you can keep track of the time.

✆ **When you're in the test room** and are about to take the actual exam, read all the directions carefully and ask any questions you have right at the top. Don't be afraid to ask.

✆ **I strongly suggest** you skim the whole test before you begin. It'll give you an overview so you'll have some sense of how to pace yourself. In terms of pacing, you shouldn't take too much time with any one question. Mark the difficult questions to go back to once you've finished the easier ones.

✆ **Some people are never clear** on whether you should guess on questions you don't know or leave them blank. The answer is to guess. A blank question is marked wrong, so you might as well take a shot at it.

✆ **Make sure** you put your name on the test booklet!

♋ **Use process of elimination.** If there are four possible answers, eliminate the ones that are obviously wrong. Then you'll be able to make a better guess between the ones that are left.

♋ **Watch out for key words** that may tip you off to "False" answers. Words like "usually," "never" or "always" are often associated with false answers.

♋ **Keep an eye out** for grammatical clues. For instance, if the last word in the clue is "an," then you know that the answer is a word that begins with a vowel ("an avocado," "an igloo," but never "an banana").

♋ **When answering true or false questions,** always remember that in order for a statement to be true, the *entire* statement has to be true.

♋ **Here's something you ought to know:** long statements are more likely to be true than short statements. Why? Because usually, you'll need enough information to prove that something is true, whereas something false can be stated in just a few words.

♋ **When it comes to multiple-choice** questions, remember that you're looking for the *best* answer. There may be other answers that are true but you need to select the best one.

♋ **If you find two choices** that both seem right, one of them must be the "right" one. Figure it out.

♋ **If one of the answers** is "all of the above," it's often the case that it's the right answer.

☙ **The best preparation** for the practical part of the exam, as far as I'm concerned anyway, are the "mock" licensing exams you'll take in school. They made all the difference for me.

☙ **Before taking the exam,** check with your regulatory agency to see if you can observe a practical examination. In some states, that's allowed.

# Taking Stock

Once you've passed your licensing examination, you can turn to the business of finding a job. A good place to start is by taking an inventory of your qualifications and interests.

☙ **My sister,** who graduated from cosmetology school a few years ago, has been my coach. She told me that when you're ready to look for a job, the first thing you should do is "grade" yourself. Make up a list of attributes—your attitude (is it positive enough?), your appearance (is it professional?), punctuality, teamwork skills, integrity and honesty, self-esteem, dependability, motivation—and honestly tell yourself whether you're "excellent," "good," "average," or "poor" in those departments. Then do the same for all the technical skills: hair shaping and cutting, haircoloring, hairstyling, texture services, makeup, and so on. When you're finished, you'll have a profile of yourself and you'll know where you have to work harder to bring yourself up to speed before you enter the job market.

☙ **No matter how good you are** at the technical stuff, the people skills are still what cosmetology is all about. Our instructor told us that success in this business depends about 80 percent on your people skills and 20 percent on your technical skills.

☙ **It's a good idea** to pick a buddy out of your class and to take turns "rating" each other on your skills. Promise to be totally, brutally honest with each other on your appearance, your attitude, your motivation, and your teamwork abilities. It might be hard to hear some of this, but in the long run, it'll be worth it.

# Regarding Résumés

A good pair of shears is a cosmetologist's basic tool and a good résumé is the basic tool of a cosmetologist in search of a job. The résumé, which is the written summary of your education and work experience, will tell potential employers at a glance all about your achievements and accomplishments. Here are some thoughts from your colleagues on the subject of résumés.

☙ **Rule number one:** Keep it short. One page. Nothing more.

☙ **Make sure** to put your résumé on good quality paper. Don't go rainbow-crazy. Maybe you think pink is your color, or orange is cheerful, but other people might hate pink or orange, so why risk it? Stick with white, buff, or gray. Okay, to you it might be boring, but to other people, it's classic.

۞ **You might have a great résumé** in terms of layout and the accomplishments you're listing, but if you don't have the necessary contact information—address, phone number, e-mail address—then what good is it going to do you? Make sure that information appears on your cover letter as well.

۞ **When it comes to résumés,** there's a big argument over how to arrange them. Check with a librarian or the Internet for format. Some people like to arrange the résumé by listing their positions chronologically, particularly if they've had significant work experience before coming to cosmetology school. Other people like to arrange it according to their accomplishments or abilities. You'll have to check it out and decide for yourself.

۞ **Use simple language.** Don't go overboard with all kinds of exaggerations. It just looks foolish.

۞ **Don't forget** to list any honors and awards you've received.

۞ **Make sure your career goals** pop out. If you're intent on doing skin care, make it clear in your résumé that that's your goal.

۞ **If cosmetology represents a career change** for you, try to convey the transferable skills you're bringing with you to this new career. For instance, if you were a manager at a clothing store in the past, pitch your managerial skills as part of your current package.

۞ **If you look at the literature** on creating résumés, they'll stress how you should always use "action verbs." You developed, achieved, created, coordinated, maintained, formulated, introduced, and so on. These words make you sound like a powerful force, which you may very well be!

☣ **Proofread, my friends,** proofread. Misspellings and poor grammar will mean points taken off. And in this competitive job market, you can't afford to lose points on stuff like that. Just ask a friend or family member to give your résumé the once-over. But make sure that person is a decent proofreader. If necessary, go back to your beauty school and draw on resources there for this task.

☣ **Nothing,** nothing, nothing goes into the résumé about your salary requirements. Could that be any clearer? Any talk about salary is restricted to your interview, and only if and when the interviewer brings the subject up.

☣ **No photos, please.** That makes your résumé look like the kind of "Most Wanted" notice you'd find in the post office.

☣ **If nothing else,** remember this rule: never, ever lie on your résumé. It will come back to haunt you, and when the grapevine gets hold of what you've done, you might have really serious problems finding a job in the town in which you live.

☣ **Some résumé reference sources** will tell you to list personal interests like hobbies or the fact that you're a member of the National Audubon Society or whatever. I've never cared for that on a résumé. Frankly, I just don't find it very relevant.

⊷ **Don't include personal references** on your résumé. It's safe to assume that everyone has someone who can speak well of her. Just list a few professional references. If a specific job asks for personal references on its job application, than that's another story.

---

## The Employment Portfolio

Another useful resource to develop for your job search is the employment portfolio. This is a collection, usually bound, of photos and other materials that exhibit your skills and accomplishments in your field. Portfolios may include any and all of the following:

✄ Diplomas, both high school and cosmetology school.

✄ Awards and achievements received while a cosmetology student.

✄ Current résumé focusing on accomplishments.

✄ Letters of reference from former employers.

✄ Summary of continuing education and/or copies of actual training certificates.

✄ Statement of membership in industry and other professional organizations.

✄ Statement of relevant civic affiliations and/or community activities.

---

- ✄ Before and after photographs of services you have performed on clients or models.

- ✄ A brief statement about why you have chosen a career in cosmetology.

- ✄ Any other information that you regard as relevant.

# Zeroing In

With your résumé in shape and portfolio assembled, you can start to target those establishments you think you might like to work in. However, keep these pointers in mind.

☾ **We all hear** a lot about "dream jobs." Don't buy into it. Dream jobs are like dream families (does anyone you know have one?). All jobs come with their problems, some worse than others. The problems are usually things like too much or too little work, crazy people, long commutes, no room for advancement, or any and all of the above. It's up to you to figure out what you think you can live with.

☾ **Let your fingers do the walking** through the *Yellow Pages*. It's a great resource and I find it a lot more "user-friendly" than the Internet. I do know some people who have found jobs off the Internet, but most people, including myself, find that it takes a long time to navigate the different sites and this time might be used more effectively otherwise.

∽ **Do we all know** by now that relying on "help wanted" ads in the newspaper is probably the least effective way of landing a good job? Many jobs are never advertised and some businesses that do advertise only run these ads because they are required to, when in fact they're really planning to promote from inside. Asking people you know is usually a far better route.

∽ **Networking** is a great way to find a job. It involves contacting people for information. For instance, you might have a cousin who knows someone who has a cousin who works for a supply house. You go through the channels and you call that person in the supply house and he might be able to put you in touch with somebody in a salon. You've networked your way into a job possibility.

∽ **I advise just calling up a salon,** if you like the looks of it, and asking if you could come in to talk. Even if there is not a job at present, it certainly won't hurt for them to know you. Most people on the other end understand that this is the way the world works and they'll probably be inclined to cooperate.

∽ **Every now and then,** your networking may end up with a door slamming in your face. If that happens, just suck it up. There are people in the world who simply aren't very nice or very helpful or very sympathetic. Don't turn the behavior of such people into a personal rejection.

∽ **When you visit a salon** that you are considering as a possibility for prospective employment, bring along a checklist to help you reach a judgment. The checklist should have questions like is the receptionist friendly and warm or not? Are waste receptacles overflowing? How are the stylists dressed? Are they wearing a uniform? If so, do you like the looks of it and would you feel comfortable wearing one? As you go from one establishment to another, keep a record of your reactions, and when you have some time, go over them and see where you're at.

☽ **A sincere "thank you"** counts for a great deal. If anyone has helped you by answering questions over the phone or by meeting with you, make sure you follow up their act of kindness with your own. A brief note of thanks will stamp you in that person's memory as someone who knows how to do the right thing.

☽ **When you call a salon** to make an appointment for an interview, you may be told they are not hiring at this time. If you're lucky, they may offer to schedule an interview with you anyway. Under no circumstances should you regard this as a waste of time. To become skilled at interviewing, you'll need a lot of practice, so seize every opportunity. What's more, maybe they'll have a look at you and think you're just right for that other job that hadn't crossed their minds!

# The All-important Interview

The résumé and the networking are designed to get your foot in the door. Okay, so now that you've got that foot in the door, what's your next step?

꙲ **When you go for your interview,** make sure, first and foremost, that you have identification with you. That means a Social Security number, a driver's license, the names and addresses of former employers, and the name and phone number of the nearest relative not living with you. Don't leave home without these!

꙲ **First impressions count** for a lot. That's just the way the world works. Think of how you've felt on occasions when a blind date comes to your door. Well, when you go into an interview, you're the blind date. That means your grooming and your wardrobe have to be spotless. An interview is no time for a halter top, no matter how hot the weather is, or jeans, or sandals, or T-shirts, or anything of the sort.

꙲ **Everything you wear** has to be clean and pressed. You are, after all, in the image industry. Your shoes have to be clean and in good repair. Keep your jewelry to a minimum (no clinky-clanky jangle bracelets, please!). And what about your hairstyle while we're at it? Is it fashionable? Does it suit your face and features? If you aren't sure, ask someone who can tell you.

꙲ **I'll let you in on a secret:** some people hate perfume. So why risk it? Leave it off that day. In fact, you might want to get out of the habit of wearing perfume altogether, because a lot of salons these days are adopting no-perfume policies.

꙲ **Carry a handbag or a briefcase,** never both. You don't want to look like you're moving in on your interviewer.

## Need a Wardrobe?

Many women find it difficult, if not impossible, to afford the two or three outfits necessary to project a confident and professional image when going out into the workplace. Fortunately, there are some wonderful nonprofit organizations that have been formed to address this need. These organizations receive donations of clean and beautiful outfits from individuals and manufacturers that are then passed along to the women who need them. For more information, check out these two web sites:

Wardrobe for Opportunity at www.wardrobe.org
Dress for Success at www.dressforsuccess.org

**Bring an extra copy** of your résumé to the interview. Even if you've already sent one, the interviewer may not have it at her fingertips, so why be caught short?

**Anticipate questions.** Obviously, you know that certain ones are going to be coming up such as "Why do you want to work here?" "What do you think you could contribute to this salon?" You need to do your homework and make sure you've got some good responses handy.

**I tell the stylists I mentor** to compile as many possible interview questions as they think they might encounter. Are you a team player? Are you flexible? What are your career goals? Are there any obstacles that would keep you from fulfilling your commitments? How would you handle a problem client? Who has influenced you most? How do you feel about retailing? Any and all of these may come up, so it helps to be ready.

☙ **Role-playing your interview** with friends or family can be very useful. Just make sure you're doing it with someone who knows how to take the charade seriously.

☙ **Some salons want you** to demonstrate a service as part of the interview. They require an applicant to bring along a model and perform a cut and style. Check to see if this is a requirement, and if it is, prepare for it.

☙ **Punctuality** is the number one rule. Never, ever, be late for an interview. Assume that if you're late, even by one minute, you've lost that job.

☙ **To make sure you don't show up late** for an interview, I advise scouting out the location a day in advance. Even if it's an hour away, make the trip and check the address. Go right up to the door so that you're not wandering around the next day in a sweat, lost in some office park when you're due for the actual interview.

☙ **Smile.** When you walk in the door, when you leave, and whenever you can in between. A good smile is one of the best tools in your tool shed.

☙ **Never lean on or touch** an interviewer's desk or place your things on the desk. Some people are very territorial and you might get marks against you for this.

☾ **Hey, people.** Don't use the interview as a time to have a coffee break, okay? Don't walk in with a cup of coffee or a can of soda or some crackers. Don't smoke or chew gum on an interview. *Puh-leese!*

☾ **Sit up straight** and speak clearly, just like your mother told you to do.

☾ **Whatever you do,** do not criticize anyone; not a teacher, not a past employer, not your Aunt Molly. An interview is not an occasion to air grievances. You'll be the one who ends up looking bad.

☾ **Always shake the hand** of your interviewer at the end and say thank you for his time.

☾ **There will come a critical poin**t in the interview when the interviewer will sit back and say, "Now, do you have any questions for me?" This is not a time to sit there, looking pretty and shaking your head no. This is a time for you to seem like an intelligent, engaged person. So come prepared with a few questions. Not a whole barrage of them; just a few well-chosen ones. For instance, you might say, "Is there a job description and may I review it?" Or "Is there a salon manual?" Maybe you want to ask what kind of opportunities there are for continuing education or if there is room for advancement. It's your call, but just be sure to have some good questions handy when the time comes.

⚭ **Don't forget to follow up** your interview with a thank-you note. It's required. And it will give you the opportunity to restate your eagerness to fill the position, which could wind up being a key factor if the interviewer is choosing between two or three people.

⚭ **Keep in mind** that there are certain questions that an interviewer does not have the right to ask and that you do not have to answer. Anything having to do with your race, religion, national origin or citizenship, age, marital status, sexual preference, disabilities, or physical traits. These are all strictly off limits. If one of these questions comes up, you should politely but firmly state that you do not think the question is relevant to the position being filled and that you would like to focus on those qualities and attributes that are relevant. The message should sink in and your interviewer may actually wind up being impressed with your presence of mind.

# Salary Negotiations

For some people, talking about money is like a trip to the dentist: they'll do anything to avoid it. But it doesn't have to be that way. Talking about money is a completely natural part of the hiring process, and you need to learn how to get comfortable with it and good at it. Here are some tips on negotiating around money.

**Do your homework.** Know what the going rate is in the neighborhood for the position being filled. The more information you have, the more powerful your negotiating position will be.

**Negotiating for a job** is not like negotiating for a car. After you buy the car, you'll probably never see the seller again. But with job negotiations, if the hiring goes through, you'll be living with the person you've been negotiating with, so it's important to operate out of good will. Keep in mind that if you're being offered the position, that means that the salon you're negotiating with has made up its mind that you're the one for the job and so you both have the same goal: to make this happen.

**Know your priorities.** If security is what races your motor, you may want more on the salary end and less on the commission end. If you're an entrepreneurial type of personality, you may want the reverse.

**There are a lot of "extras"** that factor into a total compensation package and you need to be aware of what they are. It could be vacation time, continuing education, flex time, or a six-month review with performance increases. Look into all of these and weigh them carefully when you're making your deal.

**Never lie.** If you've got a job history already, never say you made more on your last job than you actually did. On the other hand, you don't have to show all your cards. In a way, salary negotiations are a little like a game of poker: a bit of bluffing may come into play. Maybe your first time doing it won't go as well as you hoped, but with practice, you may wind up winning a few hands.

🌿 **Bargaining is expected,** but there comes a time when you run the risk of overkill. When you feel the offer is in the zone, back off. Don't hold out for every last penny. Even if your demands are met, your employer may walk away from the experience feeling that he has hired a prima donna. Remember that negotiation is about give-and-take all around.

This is an exciting time in your life. You're launching yourself on a career that can bring so much to you. You're looking forward to a good and stable income, interesting new relationships with people, an outlet for your creativity, and an opportunity to make your clients feel good about themselves. It's a wonderful career you've chosen. Now go for it!

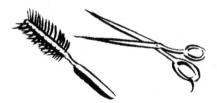

# Index

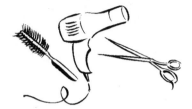